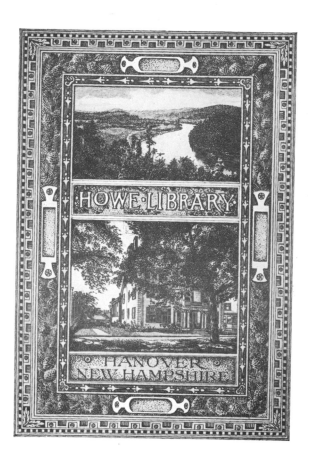

SCIENCE CATCHES THE CRIMINAL

SCIENCE
CATCHES THE
CRIMINAL

Wyatt Blassingame

ILLUSTRATED WITH PHOTOGRAPHS

DODD, MEAD & COMPANY

NEW YORK

For Alice, with love

ILLUSTRATION CREDITS: The illustrations that appear are used through the courtesy of the following: Bell Telephone Laboratories, Incorporated, numbers 11, 12, 13; Federal Bureau of Investigation, United States Department of Justice, numbers 2, 3, 4, 6, 7, 8, 9; George G. Harrap & Company, London, numbers 15, 16; Copyright © 1959 by Sir Sydney Smith. From the book MOSTLY MURDER, published by the David McKay Co. Inc. Reprinted with permission from the publishers, numbers 1, 5, 10, 14; *Punch* Magazine, London, number 17.

Library of Congress Cataloging in Publication Data

Blassingame, Wyatt.
    Science catches the criminal.

    SUMMARY: Illustrates through case histories the increasingly important role of science in the detection of crime.
    1. Criminal investigation—Juvenile literature. 2. Chemistry, Forensic—Juvenile literature. 3. Medical jurisprudence—Juvenile literature. [1. Criminal investigation. 2. Chemistry, Forensic] I. Title.
    HV8073.8.B55   364.12   75-11979
    ISBN 0-396-07152-X

CONTENTS

1

FORENSIC SCIENCE

How Did He Die?

A train rounding a sharp curve at night smashed into an automobile that exploded into flames. When the police arrived they found a man's body in the wreck, burned and mangled beyond recognition. The train's engineer had caught only a split-second glimpse of the car before it struck; yet it had seemed to him the car was already afire.

Was the body in the car that of the owner? Had his car caught fire before or after hitting the train? And had the man been killed in the accident, or was the body that of some unknown person who had been murdered elsewhere and set afire to prevent identification?

A young couple engaged to be married the very next day were found sitting side by side on the girl's living room sofa. Both were dead. But both had been in perfect health an hour before. There was no sign of violence, and no one else had been in the room. How then had they died? Was

1

it murder and suicide? A double suicide? A double murder? And how?

Both these were cases for an expert in forensic medicine.

The term forensic medicine refers to that intricate and fascinating field where medicine and the law come in contact. It does not of necessity deal with crime—if the body in the automobile was that of the owner and he had simply been killed in the accident, there was no crime. But first the body had to be identified, and the cause of death determined.

In many—perhaps a majority of—forensic medicine cases there is at least the possibility of crime. Indeed, the whole case may turn on the decision "How did the victim die?" Was it a heart attack, or a natural death; or was it murder by poison, strangulation, or how?

Medicine is not the only forensic science. Some are comparatively mechanical, such as the study of fingerprints and ballistics. Some are extremely complicated, such as the study of the types of blood and body serums, a science where new information is being gained continually. Some are ancient yet scientifically uncertain, such as graphology, the study of handwriting. Others are still in their infancy, like the use of psychiatry to guess at the physical appearance, habits, and clothing of an unknown mad murderer.

This book deals with the use of various sciences in solving—and sometimes failing to solve—crimes from around the world.

2

THE STORY OF
IDENTIFICATION

This Is Your Criminal—or Is It?

Dr. Sydney Smith, Principal Medico-Legal Expert for the Egyptian Department of Justice, was at his desk in Cairo when a police official brought in a small cloth bag. The official placed the bag on Smith's desk and then, very carefully, took out two objects. One was a worm, a very little worm, and quite dead. The other object at first glance looked as though it might have been a piece of dirty and crumpled cellophane,

"What have we here?" Smith asked.

"I—I'm not sure," the policeman said. "First, let me tell you where and how we found them."

"Go ahead."

"About two months ago we began to hear rumors that a couple, Hassan Mohammed and his wife Halima, had disappeared. They had been visiting with friends named Zenab, and then just vanished. The Zenabs said Hassan and his wife had decided to go to another town, taken their things with them, and left. But nobody's seen them since. Hassan's relatives believe he and Halima were murdered."

Dr. Smith looked more carefully now at the wrinkled object in front of him. While the policeman talked, Smith began, very cautiously, to smooth it out.

"About a week ago," the police official was saying, "a boatman reported that he'd seen a human foot sticking out of the bank of the canal. We sent some men to investigate, and they dug up the remains of two bodies. They were in very bad condition."

Smith nodded at the thing on his desk. "Is this part of it?"

"No. Or rather, that's part of our problem," the official said. "We were able to identify the bodies. They were those of Hassan and his wife all right. And they had been murdered by having their skulls crushed. But were they killed at Zenab's? Or had they actually left there and were killed elsewhere by someone else?"

Smith waited, and the policeman said, "We went through Zenab's house inch by inch. And didn't find anything. But in his garden there was a spot where the earth smelled of rot. The ground looked as if something had been buried there, then dug up again. So we dug, but these"—he pointed at the worm and the wrinkled object on Smith's desk— "were all we found."

"And if you can prove these are parts of the bodies you found, then you can prove that Hassan and his wife were killed by Zenab. If you can't show that, you have no proof?"

"That's right."

"I'll have to show the worm to a helminthologist, an

expert on worms," Smith said. "But it looks like a common roundworm, of the type that infest human intestines."

"Dr. Bey, your assistant, has already seen the bodies. He said that Hassan was infested with roundworms."

"And so are several million other persons; so that's no real proof Hassan was ever buried in Zenab's garden." Smith was looking at the other object now, still cautiously smoothing it with his fingers. "This appears to be epidermis—the very thin, outer layer of skin—of a human hand."

"Dr. Bey thought so."

"Then perhaps we can match the fingerprints with those of the body."

The policeman shook his head. "The bodies had been in the ground for three months, maybe longer. Hassan's hands are still intact, but—but barely. The woman's body has one hand missing completely. Dogs, some kind of animal, have been at it. And the other hand . . . You couldn't possibly take prints from it. Not the shape it's in."

At this time, in the mid 1920's, fingerprints were in use by most of the major police departments of the world. By now it had been proved that the tiny looped and whirled lines on the ends of an individual's fingers were formed even before birth, and they remained, absolutely unchanged, until death and at least for awhile afterward. It had also been shown that the fingerprints of no two persons were the same. But there were still things about fingerprints that many persons, including some police, did not know. The lines that look so fragile are not confined to the outer skin. Actually they are formed from the dermis, the underlying skin. And this dermis may hold the lines even after the outer skin has been stripped or rotted away.

"Where are the bodies?" Smith asked.

"Dr. Bey had them taken to your laboratory."

"All right. I'll see what I can do."

In the laboratory Dr. Smith carefully washed the bit of skin that had been brought to him. Then it was placed in Formalin to harden. While this took place he examined the remains of the woman's body.

The right hand and forearm were completely gone. The left hand remained, and it was a left hand from which the epidermis now hardening in Formalin, had come. To the naked eye the hand seemed no more than a chunk of rotting meat. But under the microscope the tiny lines—the same lines that had formed before the woman's birth—were still visible.

These lines matched exactly those of the epidermis when it was taken from the Formalin.

"And there," said Smith, "is your absolute proof that this body was once buried in Zenab's garden. And that should convict your murderer without trouble."

In the 1920's there were many things about fingerprints that only experts in forensic medicine like Dr. Sydney Smith understood. But there were also many things still to be learned, even by the experts. The story of fingerprinting is long and strange.

The very basis of all criminal justice must be the correct identification of the criminal, and of his crime. Fingerprinting is only one method of making such identification. As such, it is part of the eternal war between science and crime—a war that began a long time ago, changes shape almost daily, and will continue into the future.

A Crook to Catch a Crook

It does not always take a crook to catch a crook—as an old saying goes—but sometimes it helps. Eugène François Vidocq was possibly the first professional detective to use scientific methods to capture and convict criminals. He was also a professional criminal himself—or had been before he turned detective. Using his knowledge of the underworld, he not only became an excellent detective, he established the French Sûreté, one of the world's first and finest scientific police agencies.

Before becoming a criminal Vidocq had been an actor, a soldier, a sailor, and a variety of other things. Then one night—this was about 1792—he got in a fight with a policeman. It was over a personal matter, about a girl they both knew. But it wound up with Vidocq in prison. This was an unjust punishment, he felt, since he had committed no real crime. At the first opportunity he stole a policeman's uniform from a jail locker, put it on, and walked out. He was recaptured, and escaped again.

Now in hiding from the police, he became a real criminal. Several times he was arrested, received short sentences, or escaped. Once he climbed to the top of a prison watchtower, so high nobody thought it needed to be guarded, and jumped from there into a river flowing just outside.

Science Catches the Criminal

During one prison sentence he was chained alongside members of the Cornus family, professional criminals who taught their children how to kill.

In 1799 Vidocq escaped again and remained free for ten years. During this time he came in contact with the police on several occasions, but they did not recognize him. There was no such thing as fingerprints or photographs, or even a written description of wanted criminals. Even so, Vidocq knew there was always a chance he would be recognized and rearrested. He did not want to go back to prison, and he was weary of running from the law.

In 1810 Vidocq made a decision. He went to the Prefect of Police in Paris and admitted his identity. Then he offered a proposition. "I know more about the criminals in Paris," he said, "than all your police put together. I've lived with them. I know who they are and how they operate. Now, if you will wipe my name off your wanted list, I'll work with your police."

Vidocq had chosen the right time for his proposition. Paris was having far more than the usual amount of crime. The police were almost helpless. And yet, the Prefect knew, he couldn't simply name Vidocq, a known criminal, as a policeman. Instead, he pretended to have him arrested. Then there was a phony escape. And once more living undercover, under an assumed name, Eugène François Vidocq became a policeman.

Soon the Paris police began to make arrests that would have been impossible before. Vidocq was allowed to hire four former criminals to help him, then twelve, then twenty. His group became known as the Sûreté, the security force, and they made life miserable for Paris' crooks.

Vidocq remembered that he himself had often escaped arrest because police who had never seen him had no way to recognize him. So now he began to keep records of the physical appearance of known criminals. These were vague at best—height, complexion, scars—but they helped.

Vidocq knew that professional criminals tended to fit into patterns. A jewelry thief usually remained a jewelry thief, a pickpocket a pickpocket. Moreover, they tended to use the same method time after time: one murderer might strangle his victims, another use a knife; a burglar might always use the same method for breaking into houses.

So Vidocq and his Sûreté kept detailed records of how each known criminal worked. The records grew into massive files. If a house was burglarized by someone breaking into a second-story window, Vidocq turned to his files. Which crooks were known as second-story men? He soon had a list to work with.

In time, more respectable and sometimes less talented men followed Vidocq as chief of the Sûreté. But his files remained. Even vague as they were, they marked the first step toward the scientific detection of crime.

The Width of a Skull and the Length of a Finger

For a full half century after the time of Vidocq the police departments of the world made no real progress in how to recognize and identify known criminals. When the next step was taken, it was again the French Sûreté.

9

Science Catches the Criminal

In 1882 one of the clerks in the Sûreté was a thin, shy young man named Alphonse Bertillon. His speech was so slow that he almost stammered, and he was so shy that people thought he was stupid.

He wasn't. As a clerk he spent his time copying down the vague descriptions of criminals and wanted persons. Height, average. Hair, brown. Scars, none. Bertillon had only to raise his head to see a half dozen men who might fit this same description. There had to be a better method, he thought.

Bertillon remembered reading somewhere that the odds were four to one against any two men being the same height. Now suppose you added another measurement, say the length of the left arm. By simple mathematics this would make the odds sixteen to one. If you added eleven measurements, the odds jumped to better than four million to one.

Bertillon presented his idea in a written report to the Prefect of Police, who thought the whole thing was absurd. But the pale, shy clerk turned out to be amazingly stubborn. He began to take some measurements on his own, and he presented his plan again. And again. Perhaps the Prefect might have been able to ignore his clerk forever; but Bertillon's father and grandfather were both famous scientists and capable of bringing pressure to bear.

Finally the Prefect called Bertillon to his office. "I'll give you three months to try out your plan," he said. "If in that time you identify one person who has been in prison before, but not recognized by the police, we'll continue the experiment. If not . . ."

The Story of Identification

It was not a fair offer, and Bertillon knew it. A great many persons passed through the police station every day. But the chance that a criminal might be brought in so that Bertillon could take his measurements, then dismissed, arrested again but not recognized, all within three months, was slight indeed.

Pure luck was with him. Two weeks before his time was up he identified a petty thief using the name Dupont as one arrested two months before under the name of Martin. So the experiment was continued. With each passing month Bertillon's technique of exact measurements identified more and more recidivistic criminals that the police, relying on their memories, had missed.

Soon Bertillon added the comparatively new invention of photography to his use of measurements. Police had used some photographs before this, but without any precise method. As a result, the pictures differed widely. Bertillon had all pictures taken in exactly the same way, front and profile, under the same light. The pictures, placed alongside the measurements—these included the length of fingers, width of skull, length of skull, and so forth—gave police a far more accurate method of identifying criminals than ever before.

Within a few years the Bertillon method was adopted by practically every major police department in the world.

There was one big problem. To be of use, the Bertillon measurements had to be exact. But the measurements were taken by many different persons. In measuring a man's head one officer might push the calipers tighter against the skull than another, or he might measure a finger a little farther back on the hand. A tiny fraction of an inch might mean the difference between one man and another.

This flaw in the Bertillon system was illustrated by one of the strangest coincidences in all history. It was an accident so unusual no one would have believed it, if it had not actually happened.

In 1903 a prisoner was brought to the federal prison at Leavenworth, Kansas. His name was Willie West and he was taken to a room to be measured and photographed, just as happened to each new prisoner. While this was being done one of the guards kept staring at him. Finally the guard said, "When did you get out of here? I thought you were still here."

"I've never been here before," the prisoner said.

"Come off it," the guard said. "I've seen you around for a year or more."

The prisoner shook his head. "You saw somebody else. I've never been in jail before."

"Now wait. Your name's Willie West?"

"Yes, sir."

"Well, I'll see if you've been here before."

He asked a file clerk to see if they had a card on Willie West. In a few minutes it was brought to him. On it was a photograph, front and profile, identical to the man in front of them. Slowly the guard began to read aloud the Bertillon measurements: height, length of little finger, length of forearm, width of head—every one of them exactly the same as those the clerk had just taken.

"Only there's one problem," the guard said, looking at the file card in his hand. "This Willie West is supposed to still be here. If he's been released or escaped, there's no record of it."

"That's one thing we can find out," the clerk said.

A few minutes later a second Willie West was brought into the room. "So much alike," the guard said later, "they couldn't tell themselves which one was which. Yet they weren't any kin. They'd never seen one another before, never even heard of one another."

It was the clerk who said, "Let's check their fingerprints."

At this time fingerprinting was new, even in federal prisons. Most small prisons made no use of it at all. There was, however, an expert at Leavenworth and he was called in.

The fingerprints of the two men were totally different. But otherwise the men were identical.

The Case of Lord Salisbury-Willoughby-Wilson and Others

The Case of the Two Willie Wests helped convince police departments that something better than either visual identification or the Bertillon method was needed. For anyone who still doubted, there was what might be called the Case of Lord Salisbury-Willoughby-Wilson and Others.

This case had begun back in 1877. A tall, distinguished looking man with handsome mustaches had stopped a woman on the street in London and inquired if she was Lady Rochester. No, she said. But she was flattered at being mistaken for a member of the nobility, and she was impressed by the gentleman's looks and his handsome clothing. They stood chatting a few minutes. He introduced himself as Lord Salisbury and in turn the woman gave her own name. Lord Salisbury asked if he might call a few days later. She said yes. He did, and before two weeks had passed Lord Salisbury had proposed and been accepted.

At this point Lord Salisbury said that his bride would need more expensive clothing than she now had, so he wrote out a large check and gave it to her. He also said she would need more handsome jewelry. So he borrowed her rings, in order, he said, to buy others the same size. He borrowed her brooch and watch so he could buy her some matching pieces.

Lord Salisbury then departed. His check bounced when the lady went to cash it. And the Lord himself never came calling again.

It was by accident that the lady later saw Lord Salisbury on the street and called a policeman. Investigation proved that his name was actually John Smith, and he had robbed at least a dozen women in exactly the same way. He was sentenced to prison for five years.

This seemed to be the end of the matter. Then, after seventeen years, a woman complained to the London police that a distinguished looking gentleman with gray hair and a gray mustache had introduced himself to her as Lord Willoughby, and had eventually made off with her rings and watch. A few weeks later another woman complained, then another. The nobleman's name was sometimes different, but his technique and looks were exactly the same.

Late on the afternoon of December 16, 1896, a woman

14

named Ottilie Meissonnier rushed up to a gray-haired man on a London sidewalk. "You!" she cried. "You give my rings back, or I'll call the police!"

The man stared at her. "I don't know what you're talking about," he said stiffly.

"Oh, yes you do, Lord Wilson. Or whoever you are."

"My name is Beck," the man said. "Adolf Beck. And I've never seen you before in my life."

He pushed past the woman, but she followed, shouting at him. He crossed the street to where a policeman was standing. "I think this woman is crazy," he said. "Anyway, I hope you will make her quit following me."

Instead, the policeman took them both to the station. Several women who had complained of being robbed by an imposter posing as an English nobleman were called. Without hesitation they identified Adolf Beck as the man. The two policemen who had arrested John Smith back in 1877 were called. They identified Beck as the same man. Then more women, ten in all, came forward to identify him.

Adolf Beck was sent to prison under the name of John Smith. He was assigned the same prison identification number given Smith seventeen years before.

Beck served a little more than four years and was released. He lived quietly in London, minding his own business. Then on April 15, 1904, he walked out of his apartment and almost bumped into a woman who suddenly began to scream at him, "You stole my jewelry!"

To Beck it must have seemed like a nightmare. He began to run. The woman ran after him, shouting. A policeman joined the chase, and once more Adolf Beck was arrested. This time five women identified him as the man who had robbed them. Once more he was sentenced to prison.

A month later an actress came to the police to say she had been swindled by an apparently wealthy nobleman using the name of Lord Salisbury. Then another actress showed up with the same story about a proposal of marriage, a bad check, borrowed rings in order to replace them with more valuable jewelry. And one day later a man using the name of William Thomas was arrested while trying to pawn the rings of both actresses.

William Thomas looked amazingly like Adolf Beck—the same size, the same gray hair and waxed mustache, the same type clothing. When the women who had "positively" identified Beck as the imposter were brought in to look at William Thomas they identified him also.

In time an investigation would prove that William Thomas was not only Lord Salisbury-Willoughby-Wilson and so forth, he was also the John Smith who had first been arrested in 1877. And Adolf Beck who had twice been arrested and convicted was completely innocent.

Early Fingerprinting

The Case of the Two Willie Wests in the United States and that of Adolf Beck in England made perfectly clear that police needed some new and better method of identification.

For two thousand years and more the fact that every

human being carried his own signature on the tips of his fingers had been common knowledge in some parts of the world. In ancient China the emperors used their thumbprints to sign state papers. Artists put their fingerprints on pictures rather than their names. In Japan home owners often put their handprints above their doors. Strangely, however, no one seems to have used fingerprints in police work. William James Herschel may have been the first to use prints in this way.

In 1860 Herschel, an Englishman, was working for the British government in India. He had seen the way Chinese and Japanese used fingerprints and the subject fascinated him. Using a hand magnifying glass, he began to study his own prints, then those of his family and friends.

For awhile Herschel considered fingerprints an interesting hobby but nothing else. However, he was having trouble with his work. Part of his job was to pay monthly pensions to Indians who had worked for the British government and retired. To Herschel most of these old Indians looked alike. Often one came and collected his money; then a few days later someone using the same name would show up. Was it the same man trying to collect twice? Or was one of them a crook trying to collect the other's money?

Herschel couldn't tell.

Eventually he hit on the idea of fingerprints. He had each man who collected money sign a dated receipt with his fingerprints.

As it worked out, Herschel rarely needed to check one set of prints against another. The mysterious picture left on the paper by the fingertips—the tiny, twisting lines of loops and whorls—frightened the Indians. Most of the frauds stopped immediately. But when an imposter did show up, Herschel spotted him immediately.

It occurred to Herschel that the method he had devised might be used in the Bengal prison to register inmates. He wrote a long letter to the prison superintendent suggesting this. The superintendent had never heard of fingerprints and the idea seems to have struck him as slightly crazy. He answered Herschel politely, but the general tone of his letter was that Herschel had been in India too long; maybe the heat was affecting him and he ought to go home for a rest.

At the same time William Herschel was fingerprinting his Indian pensioners, another Englishman named Dr. Henry Faulds was working in a Japanese hospital. He saw the use the Japanese made of fingerprints and began to study the matter himself. Before long he became a little fanatical on the subject and even the Japanese laughed at his interest.

Luck gave Dr. Faulds a chance to prove it was no laughing matter. A thief broke into his neighbor's house, and in climbing over a whitewashed wall he left an excellent set of sooty handprints. A day or so later the Japanese police arrested a man they thought was the thief. Dr. Faulds asked permission to compare his prints with those left on the wall. To everybody's surprise, they were not the same.

A few days later the real thief was caught. His prints were identical with those on the wall. And Dr. Faulds became the first man to use fingerprints to free an innocent suspect.

18

The Story of Identification

In 1880 Dr. Faulds wrote an article for the British magazine *Nature* telling about his work. The police departments of the world pretty much ignored it. But it fascinated a number of men with scientific and mathematical interests. Other articles about fingerprinting began to appear. Here and there police read them with growing interest.

One of those who read the articles was Juan Vucetich in Argentina. Vucetich was using the Bertillon system, but after reading about fingerprinting he began to experiment. Soon he was so interested in the subject he went to examine the mummies in the La Plata Museum. To his delight he found the tiny lines still on their fingers, thousands of years after embalming.

Vucetich began to lecture his detectives about fingerprints. Some of them merely shook their heads, but a few listened. And one of them, named Alvarez, became the first police officer ever to use fingerprints to solve a murder.

In July of 1892 a report reached Detective Alvarez that two children had been murdered in a small village. According to the report, the mother of the children was accusing an old man who lived nearby. The old man denied it, and there was no proof one way or the other.

Alvarez went to the village. It was no more than a dozen or so dirty shacks scattered along a country road. Here Alvarez talked to the policeman who had first investigated the murder.

"The mother of the children," the policeman said, "is named Francisca Rojas. She's about twenty-six years old.

19

According to her story an old man named Velasquez has been wanting to marry her."

"Where's the father of the children?" Alvarez asked.

The policeman shrugged. "Who knows? He left here two, maybe three, years ago. Maybe they were never married. Anyway, Francisca now says she's planning to marry a young man from the next village."

"And old Velasquez?"

"There's the trouble. Apparently he's given Francisca money at one time or another. He admits he wants to marry her. She says that when she told him she was going to marry someone else, he swore he'd kill her first. She didn't take him seriously. But the next day when she came home from work she saw him leaving her house. She went in to find her two children—the oldest one was only six—dead. Their skulls had been bashed in. But we've never found the weapon."

"Then she didn't actually see him kill the children?"

"No. But she swears he must have done it. And he swears he couldn't, he was at a neighbor's house a mile down the road."

"What does the neighbor say?"

"That Velasquez was there—at the same time Francisca says she saw him leaving her house."

"So somebody is lying," Alvarez said.

He went to talk with Velasquez, then with the old man's friend. Both stuck to their story: the old man had been a mile from Francisca's home at the time she claimed to have seen him.

Alvarez called on Francisca. The house had only two

rooms with dirt floors, filthy. In one corner was the bed where the children had been murdered. The dirty sheets were still matted with blood. Francisca began to weep loudly as she pointed to the bed. "They were lying here," she sobbed. "Side by side." She put one hand over her face and turned to lean against the door with the other.

It was at this time that Alvarez saw the bloody handprint on the door. It was a gray-brown now, but still obviously blood. "The killer," he said aloud, "had to open that door, his hands still wet with the children's blood." He turned to the local policeman. "Fetch old Velasquez. Also an ink pad, some paper, and a magnifying glass."

The old man was brought. He, the policeman, and Francisca all stared curiously while Alvarez took the print of Velasquez' hand, then compared the lines of the fingers with those on the door. After awhile he turned to Francisca. "Now you."

She began to tremble. "Why? I don't understand."

Alvarez took her hand, pressed it on the ink pad, then on the paper. He studied it under the magnifying glass. He was no expert, but the lines were clear. "You murdered your own children," he said to Francisca.

For a long moment she stared at him. "Yes," she said finally. "Juan would not marry me while I had the children. He did not like them. And so . . ." Once more she began to weep.

This first case in which fingerprints were used to solve a murder illustrated another great advantage this method of identification had over that of Bertillon: a criminal was not likely to leave his exact measurements—the width of his skull and so on—behind him at the scene of his crime. But there was a good chance that he, or she, might leave finger-prints. Indeed, there have been times when the criminal left more than prints.

One of these times occurred in Pittsburgh in August, 1926. A man carrying a small cloth bag stepped up to the bank window and handed the teller a note. It read: "Don't set off the alarm, make any noise, or I'll blow up the bank. I have a bomb in my bag. Put $2,000 in small bills in a paper bag and hand it to me."

The teller read the note, and looked at the small, ugly man in front of him. He decided the man was a nut, prob-ably harmless, and stepped on the alarm button at his foot. The bank was filled with the clang of bells. A bank guard began to run toward the little man at the window, drawing his gun. The man dropped his bag—and the entire bank building shook with the terrific explosion.

When the dust settled the bank guard and the would-be robber were both dead, twenty-three other persons were injured. The robber himself had been blown to bits. Only one ear and his right hand were recognizable. But prints could be made from the right hand and these identified the robber as Robert Chowick, with a criminal record that went back at least eleven years.

A far less tragic case and one with a twist of macabre humor occurred at almost the same time in Cairo, Egypt. A burglar broke into the second story of a house where a woman lived alone. She awoke to see a dark figure leaning over her, and began to scream. The burglar clapped a hand over her mouth, but she was turning, moving her head;

his hand slipped and one finger went inside her mouth. The lady quit screaming and bit down. She bit so hard, she bit the end of the burglar's finger completely off.

The burglar fled. The woman, luckily, did not swallow the fingertip but saved it for the police. It was brought to the same Dr. Sydney Smith who had once taken fingerprints from a half-rotted epidermis.

At that time the fingerprint files of the Cairo police were still comparatively small. But Vidocq's old method of classifying criminals by their *modus operandi*, the method in which they work, was (and still is) helpful. Dr. Smith began to compare the lines on the bitten-off fingertip with the prints of known second-story burglars. And before long he knew his man.

Arrested with one finger heavily bandaged, the burglar shook his head woefully. "I think I've suffered enough losing a finger," he told the police. "I shouldn't have to go to jail too."

But he did.

Fingerprinting Today

As fingerprints were used by more and more police departments, it became obvious that some method of classifying or indexing the prints was absolutely necessary. If the New York or London or Paris police department fingerprinted every criminal arrested, then certainly their print files were going to become enormous. And if the prints left by a burglar had to be compared, one at a time, with ten or twenty thousand others, it would take years plus an army of experts to make the identification.

One of the first men to try to solve the problem was the Argentine police inspector Vucetich. About that same time an English biologist named Francis Galton devised a method. Another Englishman, Sir E. R. Henry, the Director of Scotland Yard, improved on Galton's method. Since then other changes have been made, but the system remains much the same.

Practically all fingerprints have what is called a delta, a triangular set of lines, and this delta serves as a starting point. The number of tiny ridges separating this delta from the core of the pattern is counted. Also, all fingerprint patterns are divided into one or more of five basic types called arches, tented arches, radial loops, ulnar loops, and whorls. Each of these, along with each standard area of the print is assigned a number or letter. When all ten fingers have been printed and analyzed the result may be published like this:

$$\frac{6 \quad\quad 0 \quad\quad 7 \quad\quad U \quad\quad 111 \quad\quad 15}{I \quad\quad 17 \quad\quad R \quad\quad\quad\quad 111}$$

The big fingerprint files, such as those of the FBI in the United States and Scotland Yard in England, now hold millions of prints. Yet when classified and run through a computer, any one of these may be found in minutes.

How well this system works was illustrated by a case in New York in 1965. A man who gave his name as Geneyro and said he came from Uruguay in South America was arrested for buying a large diamond ring with a bad check. His fingerprints were taken but there was no record of them in this country or in Uruguay. After he returned the ring, the police decided it would be cheaper and easier to send him back to Uruguay than keep him in prison. But just before he was released, someone suggested that his fingerprints be checked with Interpol, the international police organization. Back came word from Italy that Geneyro was actually Emilio Manero and that he was wanted for a dozen assorted crimes throughout Europe. In fact, Manero's arrest helped European police break up one of the biggest counterfeiting rings in all history.

Unfortunately, the current system of classifying fingerprints requires a complete set of all ten fingers. There is not yet a really good system of classifying single prints. If a killer leaves only one print on the trigger of his gun, the police have no way of quickly identifying this print, even if it is in their files. But scientists are now trying to invent a method whereby every single print may be reduced to a mathematical formula. Then even a single print might be run through an electronic scanner, and plucked out of millions of others within a few hours.

The more that fingerprints have been used and studied, the more has been learned about them. One expert has said that so many variations are possible that only once in 4,660,377 centuries would two person have identical prints. It's doubtful if anyone will ever be able to prove this, but certainly no two prints have yet been found alike.

At one time it was thought that these individual loops and whorls occurred only on the tips of the fingers. Now it is known they are on all "frictional skin"—the skin on the inside of the fingers, the palms of the hands, the soles of the feet, wherever the skin comes in frequent and rough contact with other objects. These other lines are just as permanent and individual as the lines on the tips of the fingers. Many hospitals now take the footprints of newborn babies so there can be no possible mix-up.

Exactly why nature placed these lines on hands and feet is not fully understood, even now. Some scientists believe they may accentuate the sense of touch. Certainly they play a part in the body's cooling system. This is done through millions of sweat pores jammed close together in the ridges that form the lines. Day and night these pour out an almost invisible mixture that is 99 per cent water, 1 per cent fatty acid. A tiny bit of this is left behind whenever the fingers touch some foreign subject. The water quickly evaporates; the fatty acid will remain, sometimes for only a few hours, sometimes for weeks. It is the trace of this oily acid that forms the fingerprint.

When police first began to use prints they merely studied them under a magnifying glass, and photographed them if possible. But such prints had to be clearly visible, like the sooty prints on a whitewashed wall left by Dr. Faulds' Japanese thief. From the first, however, scientists realized there must be prints that were often invisible. A perfectly clean finger touching a piece of paper or wood would leave traces of the oil that oozed from the pores along the ridge lines. And since any person tends to sweat more in times of nervous tension, then the burglar breaking open a window, the murderer gripping his gun, would surely leave prints.

26

These were called latent prints, and the problem was to make them visible.

The first, and still one of the most common, methods used by police was simply dusting with powder. The powder used was in contrasting color to the background. If the prints were on white paper, then a dark powder was used; if they were on dark wood, a white powder was used. This was simply dusted lightly over the surface, then blown or very carefully brushed away. The powder touching the lines of fatty acid would stick to it, and these lines could then be photographed.

This method was not too successful on rough or porous surfaces. Police now sometimes use a method called "iodine fuming." For this they need a glass tube containing iodine crystals and calcium chloride separated by a bit of glass wool. At one end of the glass tube is a small rubber hose, at the other a nozzle. The operator blows through the hose; his breath passes over the iodine crystals and the calcium chloride, and comes out of the nozzle as an iodine vapor. This can be sprayed on the surface being searched. The fatty acid of any fingerprints will absorb the iodine and turn brown. This brown will fade after a few minutes, but it lasts long enough for the prints to be photographed.

Another method uses a silver nitrate solution. This is lightly washed over the surface being studied. The silver nitrate combines with the salt in the sweat of the prints, and turns dark. Many experts now think the iodine vapor method the best of all, since it will not brush or wash away even the faintest trace of a print.

As police extended their use of fingerprints, criminals in turn tried new and sometimes desperate methods to confuse the system. It proved easy enough to avoid leaving prints—if plans could be made ahead of time. The burglar might wear gloves, the bank robber simply cover his palms and fingers with nail polish. But a hunted criminal was always in danger of being arrested on some minor charge, or even on suspicion. Then his prints, once they were on record, were an absolute identification.

Toward the end of the prohibition era in the United States there was a tremendous wave of organized crime. Gangs took on almost military organization. They waged war between themselves for the profits of illegal liquor. They staged bank robberies, kidnappings, and jail breaks. Many of the leaders were well known to the police, but catching them was something else. They used disguises, hideouts, moved from one part of the country to another. But the lines on their fingers went with them and could not be disguised.

Or could they?

In January, 1934, Chicago police got a tip that a gangster called Pretty Jack Klutas was hiding in a small house in one of the suburbs. As they closed in, Pretty Jack decided to shoot his way out. Instead, he was killed. Even though he was now dead, his fingerprints were taken as a matter of record—and the police got a shock. There were no lines on the tips of Pretty Jack's fingers. The fingertips were white, a little raw looking, and perfectly smooth to the naked eye.

A doctor was called in. He examined the hands of the corpse and smiled sourly. "He's had a doctor working on him. A crooked doctor, but one good at his job. All the skin has been peeled from his fingers. Even so—" the police doctor shrugged, "it couldn't have done him any good. If he'd lived long enough for the skin to grow back, it would have had the identical lines it always had. Look carefully and you can see where they are already beginning to form."

The most famous of all the outlaws of the 1930's was John Dillinger. Wanted for a variety of murders, bank robberies, and kidnappings, Dillinger, like Pretty Jack, was hiding out in Chicago and wanted to change his fingerprints. Two doctors were brought to his hideout to work on him. But it turned out that Dillinger was allergic to the anesthetic used. He almost died before there was time to operate. When he recovered, Dillinger grabbed a machine gun and threatened to kill the doctors. After that they decided to be more careful. They used acid to burn away the skin of the fingertips, bit by bit.

Recovering from the burns, Dillinger grew restless in his hideout. One night he decided to go to a movie. As he came out, the police (once more they had been tipped off by some member of the underworld) closed in. Dillinger tried to draw a gun. Perhaps his hands were still sore. Anyway, he did not draw fast enough and was killed.

When fingerprints were taken from his corpse the lines were already beginning to reform—exactly the same lines he had been born with, and had died with.

It is now known that there is only one way permanently to remove the telltale lines from fingertips—short of cutting off the fingers. It has been done at least once, by a crooked doctor working on a professional criminal.

In the fall of 1941 a Texas Highway Patrolman saw a

man hitchhiking just outside Austin. The officer stopped to question him, merely as a matter of routine. The hitchhiker, a slender, rather good-looking young man, said he was on his way to the West Coast looking for a job. His name, he said, was Robert Pitts. At this time all young men were required to carry military draft cards. Asked to show his, Robert Pitts fumbled around, then said he'd lost it. As he searched for the draft card, the patrolman noticed that his fingers had an odd, abnormally smooth look.

The patrolman took Pitts to headquarters on a charge of traveling without a draft card. He was fingerprinted, and the fingerprint expert stared in disbelief at the ink stains on the paper. There were no loops nor whorls nor arches. There were no lines at all.

Robert Pitts simply grinned and said his fingers had always been that way.

A man without lines on his fingers was far more fascinating to police than a man without a draft card. Pitts was tucked away in jail on the draft card charge, and photographs of his lineless prints were sent to the giant FBI file in Washington. The FBI consulted with various medical experts, then telephoned the Austin police to search Pitts' body for scars.

On each side of Pitts' chest there were five oval scars. If he held his arms folded across his chest, then the tips of his fingers fitted exactly over the scars.

Some crooked doctor had removed the skin from Pitts' fingers. Then patches of skin had been removed from his sides. His arms folded across his chest, his fingers had been taped to his sides until new skin from his sides grew onto his fingers. Such a skin graft, the doctors said, could be made only with skin from his own body. It could not create a new set of fingerprints; but it did replace the old skin with smooth, nonfriction skin from his sides.

Why would any man go through such a painful operation to remove his fingerprints? The answer was obvious: he was wanted by the law and was trying to avoid identification. So now Pitts' picture and description were sent to every police department in the country. Quite soon he was identified as Robert Phillips, known to his underworld pals as Roscoe. He was a specialist in safe blowing, and was wanted for three jobs along the East Coast.

Roscoe-Pitts-Phillips went back to prison, still boasting that his fingertips were as unlined as a baby's bottom. Which they were. But being without lines on his fingertips was far more unique than being without a draft card. And this was exactly the reason the police had been so determined to learn his identify.

3

THE STORY OF
BALLISTICS

The Innocent Found Guilty

It was barely daylight, March 22, 1915, when Charles Stielow got out of bed. He put new wood on the fire in the small stove, then stood close to it while he dressed. Pulling on a heavy jacket he opened the door and went out.

At the foot of his front steps lay the body of a woman. She wore only a nightgown, and the gown, the woman's head and face were thick with clotted blood.

For a full half minute Charles Stielow simply stood and stared down at the body. He was a huge man, still young, powerful, kindly, but with the mind of a child. He had never before seen a dead person. Now he simply stood and looked until he realized, slowly, that the woman was Margaret Wolcott, housekeeper for the old farmer for whom Charles Stielow worked.

It had snowed during the night. A trail of blood was plainly visible from the body toward the farmer's house some two hundred feet away. Charles Stielow followed it up the rear steps to the open door.

Inside the door lay Charles Phelps, the seventy-year-old farmer. He too wore a nightgown, the chest splotched with blood.

Stielow went slowly back to his cottage. He awakened his brother-in-law, Nelson Green, told him what he had seen, and asked him to go for the sheriff.

When the sheriff and two deputies arrived it was quickly obvious that the killer, or killers, had broken into Phelps' home intending to rob the place. Drawers had been pulled out, a desk broken open. Apparently Phelps had heard them, come to see what was happening, and been shot. Then the housekeeper had heard the noise. She had been smashed over the head, but had run as far as Stielow's cottage before dying.

This was in a rural area of New York State where crimes were few. Sheriff Bartlett brought in a bloodhound, but on the frozen snow the hound found no scent. By this time, word of the murders had spread and curious neighbors had trampled over any tracks left by the killers.

An autopsy produced three bullets from Phelps' body. They were all .22 caliber. In the year 1915 this was about all anyone could tell about used bullets.

Old man Phelps had been popular in the neighborhood and Sheriff Bartlett felt he had to do something about the crime. Trouble was, he didn't know what. But the two easiest persons to suspect were Charles Stielow and his brother-in-law Nelson Green.

At first Stielow could not understand why the sheriff

kept asking him questions. He'd told all he knew. Then he became frightened. He stumbled over his answers. No, he said, he didn't have a .22 gun. He didn't have a gun of any kind.

Nelson Green was, if anything, more stupid than Stielow. The sheriff and deputies went to work on him. For hour after hour they kept at him. If he didn't confess, they said, he would surely go to the electric chair. If he did confess, they would let him off lightly. He could put the blame on Stielow. He could say it was all Stielow's idea.

Terrified, Green told them that his brother-in-law did own a .22 pistol. The sheriff and deputies continued their third degree of Green, keeping him without food or sleep. Before long, totally confused, he was willing to agree to anything. He would sign any confession they wrote for him—except that he could neither read nor sign his own name.

Now the sheriff turned to Stielow again. Faced with Green's "confession," Stielow admitted he did have a .22 pistol. He showed the officers where it was hidden. But he would not confess having killed Phelps.

It took the sheriff and deputies two days of steady questioning. But at last the huge, slow-witted man broke. He would agree to anything, even that he had killed Phelps, if they would just leave him alone.

When Stielow was brought to trial he repudiated his confession and told how he had been forced to make it. Also, the confession had holes obvious to anyone who would stop to look. If Stielow and Green were the killers, why had Margaret Wolcott run toward their house instead of away from it after being attacked? Why had they left her body lying on their front doorstep?

These questions did not bother the prosecuting attorney. He had the three .22 caliber bullets taken from Phelps' body, and he had Stielow's .22 caliber gun. Moreover, he had something quite new in forensic science; he had an "expert," who could prove, he said, that the bullets came from Stielow's gun.

This "expert" was a man named Dr. Albert Hamilton. He had awarded himself the title of doctor while selling patent medicine. Now he was advertising himself as an expert in "chemistry, microscopy, handwriting analysis, toxicology, identification of bloodstains, causes of death, embalming, anatomy, gunshot wounds, guns, identification of bullets, gunpowder, and high explosives." His services were for sale to either side of a question that had the money to pay him. Charles Stielow had no money, but the prosecution did.

Although Hamilton's claim to be an expert on anything was as phony as his title of doctor, he was, in fact, a remarkable man, well ahead of his time. In 1915 there were practically no true experts in "identification of bloodstains . . . identification of bullets . . . gunshot wounds" anywhere in the world. Indeed, there were very few persons, even among law enforcement officers, who understood how important such an expert would be.

Hamilton fetched a mircroscope and several large, very blurred photographs to the courtroom. These were pictures of the bullets taken from Phelps' body, he said. And each bullet had a scratch on it, he said, that exactly matched a scratch in the barrel of Stielow's gun. When Stielow's lawyer pointed out that the pictures did not show any scratch, Hamilton replied that he'd brought the wrong pictures: these were of the *other* side of the bullets.

The jury found Charles Stielow guilty and sentenced him to the electric chair.

Fortunately, before Stielow could be executed, another man, arrested on a totally different charge, confessed to the murder of Phelps and Margaret Wolcott. His story fitted the details perfectly. But then he changed his story and said he'd had nothing to do with the killing.

What followed was a public uproar. Some newspapers took one side, some the other. The governor of New York appointed a commission to investigate and find the truth.

One member of this commission was a man named Charles Waite. He was middle-aged, in poor health, and up to this time he'd never had any great interest in guns. But now he was faced with a situation in which a man's life depended on whether or not three small pieces of lead had come from a certain gun.

Charles Waite went hunting for the best experts available. He talked with gunsmiths, police officers, scientists. He did not have a microscope; he didn't even know how to look through one; so he took the bullets to an optical company. There a microscopist, peering carefully at the bullets, said they showed no such scratch as Albert Hamilton had described.

Waite fired Stielow's pistol into a box of wadded cotton, and turned these bullets over to the microscopist. They showed no such scratch either. The scratch had been a figment of Hamilton's imagination.

What all the bullets did show under the microscope were fine, spiraling lines with grooves between them. A gunsmith explained to Waite that the barrel of a rifle or pistol was made from a solid block of steel. Through this steel a hole is bored by automatic cutters, working in an oil bath. These cutters left tiny ridges, called lands, with grooves between them. The lands and grooves went in a spiral and a bullet passing through the barrel would begin to spin with them. It would then travel faster and straighter than a bullet that came from a smooth bore gun. A bullet from a smooth bore gun would soon begin to tumble in flight and curve.

Practically all manufacturers of pistols and rifles used spiral bores. But in some brands of guns the lands and grooves turned to the right, in some to the left. Some of the spirals were much tighter than others.

Examined under the microscope it was obvious that the bullets from Stielow's pistol and those from Phelps' body had not come from the same brand of gun. After three years in prison, Charles Stielow was given a pardon.

For Charles Waite, however, the Stielow case was only a beginning. By now he had become totally fascinated with guns and with the identification of bullets. If such knowledge had saved one man's life, it might save many others as well as convict the guilty. Waite got his own microscope. He began to visit one gun factory after another. He collected data on practically every make of gun in the United States.

Then a police officer told Waite that two-thirds of the guns used by criminals in the United States were made abroad. He went abroad and spent a year going from one gun factory to another. By 1926 he was able to peer through his microscope at almost any bullet and tell what type of gun had fired it.

This was a tremendous advance in the science of ballistics, but it fell far short of what was really needed. Waite could examine a bullet and know it had been fired by, say, a Colt .32 caliber pistol. He might even be able to say that this particular pistol had been manufactured somewhere between 1915 and 1924. But in that time Colt would have made literally thousands of .32 caliber pistols.

Was there any way to determine not just the brand of gun that fired a particular bullet, but the exact individual gun itself?

A gunsmith told Waite that this should be possible. "You look at a razor blade with the naked eye," the gunsmith said, "and they all look alike. The edge is smooth, sharp; that's all you can see. But under a microscope you'll see that actually that blade isn't smooth at all. There are nicks, gaps, jagged edges. And every time you shave these change just a little. Now the automatic cutters boring their way through the barrel of a gun—they have nicks and cuts and rough edges also. And these change with every barrel bored. So every single gun barrel must leave what you might call individual fingerprints, if you examine the bullets carefully enough, under a microscope that's powerful enough."

One other thing was needed, Waite decided. Under his microscope he could examine one bullet at a time. To compare it with another he had to hold the memory of the first in his mind. And human memory was fallible. He needed a microscope under which he could compare two bullets at the same time.

Charles Waite never perfected such a microscope. In 1926 he died of a heart attack. But by then he had inspired several scientists to join him in establishing the Bureau of Forensic Ballistics, the first institute of its kind in the world. Also, the New York police had become extremely interested in this new science. And in Cairo, Egypt, another man who knew little or nothing of Charlie Waite was working on the same problem.

The Murder of the Sirdar

In the first part of this century Egypt was under the control of the British government. In their struggle for independence Egyptian extremists began a series of political murders, killing both British and Egyptian officials. Any bullets that were found in the bodies of the victims were sent to Dr. Sydney Smith, the forensic science expert for the Egyptian government.

It was in 1919 that Dr. Smith first began seriously to study these bullets and to learn all he could about the science of ballistics. He knew that back in 1835 a murder had been solved by a study of the bullet. But this had been a handmade bullet with a very obvious pimple on it; the police had been able to match it with a mold owned by one of the suspects. So far as Smith knew, little, if anything, had been added to the science of ballistics since then.

Like Charles Waite, Smith soon realized that he needed

a microscope that would let him compare two bullets at the same time. Scientifically trained, he managed to develop one of his own. (Later the New York Police Department would develop vastly improved comparison microscopes such as those in use today.)

Using his comparison microscope, Smith quickly learned that the bullets used in the various assassinations had nearly all come from a small number of guns. One gun in particular had been used over and over. Following Charles Waite's method of counting the grooves (there were six) and noting the angle, Smith felt sure the gun was a .32 Colt automatic. He also felt sure he would have no trouble identifying this particular gun, if he could ever find it. Each bullet was distinctly marked by a scratched groove that must have been made by a fault near the muzzle end of the barrel.

The problem was how to find this gun.

It was probably an old gun, Smith decided, because of the flaw in the barrel. In fact, a careful study of all the bullets indicated that most of them came from old guns. Because so many of them came from the same guns, Smith believed the political murders were all being done by a small group of men. It was possible they kept all their guns hidden in the same place, then took them out when needed.

In November, 1924, in broad daylight, occurred the most spectacular of all the murders.

Sir Lee Stack Pasha, the Sirdar (Commander-in-Chief) of the Egyptian Army was riding in a chauffeur-driven car through the middle of Cairo. With him was his aide-decamp. On one of the busiest streets of the city the automobile slowed to avoid a streetcar. At this instant the assassins struck. From both sides of the street men ran toward the automobile, firing pistols. Everyone in the auto was hit, but somehow the chauffeur kept driving. The killers ran after the car, still firing.

As the Sirdar's car sped away, one of the assassins turned and threw a bomb back into the crowd. It did not explode, but in the confusion the assassins jumped into a taxi they had waiting and escaped. Next day the Sirdar died of his wound.

As usual, the evidence was brought to Dr. Smith. This time it consisted of six bullets taken from the bodies of the victims, and nine cartridge cases found on the street. Five of the bullets had cross marks cut in the tips. The purpose of the cuts was to make the bullets expand when they struck some object, and in that way make a larger, more deadly wound.

One of these—the bullet that had actually killed the Sirdar—came from a Colt .32 with a flaw near the muzzle.

By now the Egyptian police were fairly sure that all the political murders were the work of a secret society. Some of the members were known, but none of these had been seen to take part in the murder of the Sirdar. There were no clues to the actual killers.

Finally an undercover policeman learned that two brothers named Enayat may have taken part in the murder. Still, there was no legal evidence against them.

"If we could catch them carrying guns," Dr. Smith told

the police, "and if those were the guns used in the murder, I could prove it by the bullets."

"But they don't carry the guns with them," the official said. "I've had men watching them secretly for days. And I'm sure they don't carry guns."

"The guns are probably hidden," Smith said. "Even if we arrested them and searched their houses, we probably couldn't find the guns. We'll have to make them find the guns for us."

"How?"

"If they thought they were going to be arrested unless they left the country, they might then try to escape, taking the guns with them."

"Maybe that can be arranged," the official said.

An undercover policeman went to the brothers, posing as a member of the secret society. He told them the police were planning to arrest and force them to confess to the murder of the Sirdar. Their only chance to escape, he said, was quickly to take the train out of Egypt to Tripoli.

The brothers took the train. But as the train was crossing a desert, it stopped. From each end of the car police closed in. They arrested the brothers, searched them—and found nothing.

It seemed that the plan had failed. Then one policeman accidentally kicked over a basket of fruit. And out fell four pistols. One of them was a Colt .32.

Now the problem was up to Sydney Smith. Was this truly the gun that had been used in the killing of the Sirdar and other political murders as well?

Dr. Smith brought in twenty-four other Colt .32s. He

had policemen fire them one after another into a box stuffed with cotton. Then the gun taken from the brothers Enayat was fired. Each bullet was numbered to match the gun that had fired it. Smith compared them, one at a time, with the bullet from the Sirdar's body.

The only one that matched was from the Enayats' pistol.

The experiment was repeated. And repeated. Each time the result was the same. There could be no doubt. The gun that had fallen from the brothers' basket of fruit was the gun that had killed the Sirdar.

Faced with this proof, the brothers confessed.

Science to the Rescue

An expert in ballistics, like any other scientist, should be totally impartial, impersonal. His purpose is not to convict, but to learn the truth—which may lead to conviction, or acquittal.

In San Francisco the night of July 8, 1964, was cool and foggy. From the Bay came the repeated, lonely sound of foghorns. In the living quarters of the Rancho Lombard Motel, Leonard Overton, the motel manager, could hear the horns even though the windows were closed against the fog. "It must be thick out there tonight," he said to his wife.

She was watching television and nodded without answering.

A few moments later the bell in the office rang. "Somebody checking in late," Overton said. He walked into the office, leaving the door to the living quarters open behind him.

Mrs. Overton was not listening to what was said in the office. But suddenly one short sentence burst into her consciousness, a man's voice saying, "This is a stickup!" It was followed almost instantly by the sound of a struggle. A gun fired.

Mrs. Overton sat motionless, unable to move. Then she was running toward the office. She saw her husband on the floor, beyond him a woman going out the door. Near the door stood a man holding a pistol. For one moment he and Mrs. Overton stared at each other. Then the man turned and vanished into the fog outside.

When the police arrived they found Leonard Overton dead, his wife in hysterics. But she was able to tell them what had happened. She'd had only a glimpse of the woman, she said. However, she'd seen the man clearly. He was about six feet tall, or taller, dark-haired. She couldn't really describe him, but she was sure she would know him, if she saw him again.

The police began a routine investigation. They compared the details of this crime with those of other holdups, hoping the *modus operandi* would point to a criminal who had used this method in the past. And they began calling in stool pigeons to ask for leads. Who had been desperate for money? Or who had suddenly got money? Who would take his girl friend with him on a holdup?

There was a quick break. An informant told the police about a couple living in a motel not far from the Rancho Lombard. They were both dope addicts and in need of money. The man, named Lawrence Camargo, was tall and dark.

The police arrested them. A quantity of heroin was found in the room. Mrs. Overton identified them. She was absolutely certain, she said, Camargo was the killer.

The police could not find the gun, but that might have been thrown away. It looked like an open-and-shut case, and the trial date was set for a few months ahead.

At this point Inspector Al Birdsall of the San Francisco police heard about another murder. Down the coast in Santa Barbara a man had just been arrested for shooting a motel owner during a holdup. He had used a .32 caliber automatic, similar to the one used in the Rancho Lombard murder.

Birdsall felt sure he had the killer from the Rancho Lombard. Still, the two cases were so much alike it might be well to investigate. He and John Williams, the police laboratory examiner, took a plane to Santa Barbara.

At the jail they quickly decided the trip had been a waste of time. The suspect was an ex-convict named Gerald Moore. But he wasn't six feet tall or taller. He was slightly under five-feet-five. Even so, Birdsall knew that human beings under the stress of great excitement can make big mistakes in judgment. Mrs. Overton might have misjudged.

John Williams fired bullets from Gerald Moore's gun and put them under a microscope alongside the bullet that had killed Leonard Overton. They did not match.

Birdsall and Williams went back to San Francisco. The time for the trial of Lawrence Camargo drew closer.

Then Inspector Birdsall got a phone call from Santa

Barbara. The police, searching Gerald Moore's home, had found another gun, another .32 automatic, hidden under a pile of old clothing. Would Inspector Birdsall like to see a test bullet from this gun?

Birdsall would. And this time John Williams, peering through his comparison microscope, matched it land for land, groove for groove, scratch for scratch with the bullet from the body of Leonard Overton.

As a result, Lawrence Camargo, who had been "positively identified" as the killer of Overton, was released. Gerald Moore was charged with the murder.

What may be the strangest case in the history of ballistics occurred in Egypt. It matched one of the most ancient of arts with what was one of the newest of sciences.

The Egyptian desert has always been a good place for murder. It is a barren land, cut sometimes by rough gulleys, sometimes by piled sand dunes. Here a would-be killer can hide until his victim is within a few yards. And since few persons travel the desert, a body may remain unfound until nothing is left but a skeleton.

In this case, in the early 1920's, the victim was found within a few days after his death. He was an Egyptian, a postman who often walked across this narrow strip of desert between one village and another. He had been killed by a bullet passing from right to left through his head. The police searched the area but did not find the bullet or any other clues to go on.

At this point, Bedouin trackers were called in by the police. These Bedouins were Arabs, nomads who had lived in the desert for generations. For them, tracking was both an art and a science. Small children were taught to recognize the tracks of their parents and of animals belonging to the family. Later they learned to recognize the tracks of friends as readily as they recognized faces. From the tracks of a stranger they could tell whether it was a man or woman, how tall, how heavy, whether running or walking.

Two of these Bedouins were taken to the spot where the dead man had been found. The police stood back to watch.

Since the police had already searched the area, there were numerous tracks. First, the Bedouins studied these, recognizing them by the type of shoes the police had worn. Then one of the trackers pointed to the ground. "This was not a policeman," he said. "This man wore sandals, not shoes."

The other Bedouin nodded. Together they followed the sandal tracks for about forty yards. There, back of a low sand dune, they found the marks where a man had knelt on the ground. "The killer fired from here," one said.

Again the other nodded. A moment later he stooped and picked up an empty cartridge case from a .303 rifle.

Once more the Bedouins followed the tracks. After firing, the killer had apparently gone to look at the body of his victim. Here he had removed his sandals and had run barefooted until he reached a dirt road. There were many tracks on the road, but still the Bedouins picked out those of the killer. They followed these until they reached a fort where members of the Egyptian Camel Corps were camped. On the paved courtyard of the fort, the tracks ended.

Next day the officer in charge of the Camel Corps marched his men across a strip of prepared sand. The

Bedouins examined the tracks—and immediately pointed to one set. "These were made by the same man we followed here," they said.

The experiment was repeated two more times. Each time the Bedouins picked out the tracks of the same man. Once more the officer marched his men across the sand, this time without the one whose tracks had been identified. The Bedouins studied the tracks. "He is not here," they said.

By now the police were sure they knew the killer. But he denied the crime; he denied even knowing the man who had been killed. And the only proof—the story of the Bedouin trackers—would not stand up in a modern court.

The bullet that had killed the postman was lost somewhere beyond finding. But the police now had the empty shell case from the .303 rifle. This was brought to Dr. Sydney Smith.

By this time Smith had learned that a shell casing bore its own type of fingerprints as exactly as did a fired bullet. The mark of the firing pin and its position on the shell might differ. The marks of the bolt, marks left by the recoil of the shell when fired, scratches from the ejector or from the chamber of the gun, might vary. All together they offered positive identification.

Dr. Smith collected the rifles of all the Camel Corps members. He also rounded up every other .303 rifle he could find locally, 53 all together. Then he fired six bullets from each, a total of 318 shells.

One by one he put them under his comparison microscope alongside the one found in the desert. And the rifle he identified belonged to the same soldier identified by the Bedouins.

Faced with this combination of ancient and modern sciences, the soldier confessed. He had killed the postman, he said, because of a quarrel over a girl—a quarrel both as ancient and as modern as the sciences which had trapped him.

4

BLOOD WILL TELL

The Mad Killer of Rügen Island

On the afternoon of September 9, 1898, a nine-year-old girl named Else Langemeier was late coming home from school. At first her mother did not worry. This was in Lechtingen, a small German village where the child knew almost everyone. She had probably stopped to play with one of her classmates, her mother thought. But as it began to get dark, the mother set out to look for her.

No one, it seemed, had seen the child since early morning. In fact, she had not reached school. Neither had one of her close friends, Hannelore Heidemann. The two children had simply disappeared. The last anyone had seen of them they had been on their way to school, their arms full of books, and talking to a man named Ludwig Tessnow.

This Ludwig Tessnow was not a native of Lechtingen. He had told someone that he came from the island of Rügen in the Baltic, but no one really knew much about him. He was a carpenter who wandered from one town to another, doing odd jobs. The few people he had worked for in Lechtingen thought he was a good carpenter, but probably simpleminded. There were times when his eyes seemed to focus on something that no one else could see. He smiled and talked to himself in a whisper.

Tessnow admitted having seen the children on their way to school. He had said good morning, commented on how many books they were carrying, then gone about his own work. That was all he knew, he said.

It was next day that the bodies of the girls were found in a nearby woods. They had been murdered, and horribly mutilated.

Suspicion quite naturally fell on Ludwig Tessnow. He was arrested, and the tumbledown shack where he lived was carefully examined. But the only bit of possible evidence was the fact that his clothes were badly stained with brown smears that might have been blood. Tessnow insisted the stains were made by a brown paint that he used in his work, and it was true that he was using such a paint.

In the year 1898 there was no one in Lechtingen who could prove or disprove what caused the stains.

The people of the town were soon divided into two camps over the question of Ludwig Tessnow's guilt. Certainly the two children had been murdered, and to all appearances the murders were the work of a madman. It was difficult for the villagers to believe that one of themselves was the killer. So it had to be Tessnow, many persons thought. Others said it was cruel and unjust to accuse a man of murder merely because he was a stranger and simpleminded. The only evidence against him was the brown stains that he claimed to be paint.

The law itself was more objective than the people of

Lechtingen. Tessnow was held in jail for several weeks. But when the police could find no real evidence against him, he was released. He walked out of the town, carrying his carpenter tools, smiling faintly, and whispering to himself.

At about the same time Ludwig Tessnow walked out of Lechtingen, a twenty-eight-year-old doctor named Paul Uhlenhuth was at work in the laboratory of the Institute of Infectious Diseases in Berlin. He was trying to find a way to immunize cattle against hoof-and-mouth disease, but he was also on the trail of an even greater discovery.

From the work of a Dr. Emil von Behring, Uhlenhuth knew that when an animal was inoculated with a very small amount of a specific toxin—the germ, or poison, that caused a specific disease such as tetanus or diphtheria—then the blood of that animal would in some mysterious way create a substance, called an antitoxin, to fight against this particular toxin. He knew too that if a rabbit was inoculated with cow's milk, the rabbit's blood would create a substance to protect it against the protein in the milk. Not only that. If serum—the liquid part of the blood—was taken from this rabbit and mixed with cow's milk, an odd thing would happen: the protein cells in the milk would agglutinate, separate from the rest of the serum and clump together. Under a microscope this was clearly visible.

This was Dr. Paul Uhlenhuth's starting point. He began by injecting the protein from a hen's egg into a rabbit. And he found that if protein from any hen's egg was mixed with that rabbit's serum, it would precipitate. But the protein from a duck egg, a goose egg, a bird egg would not precipitate. So there must be a difference, he thought, between the protein in the egg of a hen and in the eggs of other fowls.

Dr. Uhlenhuth began to work with hen's blood. He found that this reacted exactly as did the protein from the egg. Serum taken from the inoculated rabbit would agglutinate when mixed with blood from a hen. It would not agglutinate if mixed with the blood of a goose.

Uhlenhuth moved now to other animals and found the same thing to be true. Serum from a rabbit that had been inoculated with the blood of a horse would agglutinate when a drop of horse blood was mixed with it. It would not agglutinate when mixed with the blood of a dog, a pig, a monkey.

And serum from a rabbit inoculated with the blood of a human being would agglutinate when mixed with the blood of a human being.

In February, 1901, Paul Uhlenhuth published a scientific paper about his findings. In it he wrote: "I have succeeded in taking blood of man, horses, and cattle dissolved in physiological NaCl [salt] and dried on a board for four weeks and in identifying the human blood at once by means of my serum—a fact that should be of particular importance to forensic medicine."

There was one small problem, Uhlenhuth noted. The blood of closely related animals could not be separated: the blood of a horse could not be told from that of a donkey; the blood of a man could not be told from that of certain species of monkeys. But in most cases this would offer no problems.

Some four months after the publication of Dr. Uhlenhuth's paper, a farmer on the island of Rügen was returning home in the early evening. Ahead of him, on the opposite side of a pasture, he saw a man running. The farmer had only a glimpse of the man; still, it struck him as if there was something odd about the person, something furtive, as if he were trying to keep from being seen.

The farmer shrugged and forgot the incident—until the next morning. At that time, recrossing the same pasture, he found something he had missed in the early darkness the day before. It was the head of a sheep—just the head.

Then a found a leg. A few yards away was another leg. A few yards from that was a pile of intestines.

Altogether six sheep had been slaughtered, hacked to pieces, and scattered about the pasture. Apparently nothing had been taken for food. The sheep had simply been slaughtered, cut into fragments, and scattered senselessly about.

It caused a sensation on the island of Rügen where sheep were an important economic part of life. The farmer told of the man he'd seen running from the pasture, but could not say who it was.

Three weeks later there was an event that made people forget the sheep. Eight-year-old Hermann Stubbe and his six-year-old brother Peter failed to come home for supper. Their father went looking for them. Then he called on his neighbors to help. But it was next morning before the children were found in a nearby wood. They had been murdered, their bodies hacked into pieces and scattered like those of the sheep.

A road worker told the police that late on the day the

Stubbe boys were killed he had seen Ludwig Tessnow in the same area. Tessnow's clothing had been stained with something that looked like blood.

The police arrested Tessnow. They found that he had two sets of clothes. One was for Sundays and holidays, the other for work. Both had a number of brown stains on them. But the stains, Tessnow said, were made by the brown paint he used in his work.

It was the talk of brown paint that reminded one of the police of the two little girls who had been murdered in Lechtingen three years before. He sent a message to those officials—and learned for the first time that the man under suspicion in that case had been Ludwig Tessnow.

Now the Rügen police felt sure they had the murderer. Still, they had no more legal proof of his guilt than had the Lechtingen police. Tessnow sat in prison smiling faintly and whispering to himself.

It was a situation that had confronted the police of many countries for many years. A man might be suspected of murder and his clothes be badly soiled with what might be blood. But if he claimed the stains were made by paint there was no way to prove him wrong. Even if the stain was so fresh as to be unmistakably blood, he might claim it was blood of some animal he'd killed.

Ludwig Tessnow had been released once. He might have been released again. But the Rügen prosecutor had read the paper published by Dr. Uhlenhuth. He sent Tessnow's two suits of clothing to the scientist.

There were nearly one hundred separate spots on the two suits. Where possible, Uhlenhuth scraped off some of the stain with a knife blade, then dissolved it in a salt solution. Where the stain was too small for this, he cut the soiled spot out of the clothing and soaked the whole thing in his solution. Then he began to check against his prepared serums.

Tessnow's work clothing showed no blood of any kind.

But on Tessnow's Sunday clothing Uhlenhuth found human blood in twenty-two different places. He also found nine spots of sheep's blood.

Ludwig Tessnow was convicted of murder and executed. He went to his death still smiling faintly and whispering to himself.

A Killer Goes Free

On the night of May 21, 1939, the police in Branksome, England, received a telephone call from a frantic-sounding young man. Come quick, he said, his grandfather had been murdered. He gave an address in a well-to-do area.

Inspector Leonard Burk of Scotland Yard answered the call. He found a large stone house set back from the road behind a beautifully kept garden. Waiting on the front step were two young people who gave their name as Dinivan. They were brother and sister, and it was their grandfather who had been murdered.

Walter Dinivan, the dead man, lay on the floor of the living room, a dark pool of blood around his head. While Inspector Burk stood quietly studying the scene, young Dinivan told his story.

He was in the Royal Navy, Dinivan said, and had only recently come home on leave. Home was his grandfather's house where his sister Hilda also lived, acting as housekeeper for her widowed grandfather. That night the two young people had gone dancing. When they came home it was still early, but the front door was locked. The living room was dark, but looking through the window they could see their grandfather by the light of the fire. He lay on the floor with something dark around his head. Young Dinivan thought his grandfather must have become sick, vomited, and passed out on the floor. He ran to the front door, broke it open, and went in to find Walter Dinivan dead, his head a bloody mess. The young man had immediately called the police, he said, and nothing in the room had been touched.

A medical examiner had arrived along with Burk. Kneeling beside the body he told the inspector, "It looks as if someone tried to strangle Dinivan from behind. When that didn't work, they hit him over the head with something, possibly a hammer. And kept hitting him. I can be more definite after the autopsy."

Burk nodded. He had already noticed that near the far wall a small safe stood open and empty. On the floor beside it was a key. "That's the key to the safe," Hilda said when Burk asked her. "Grandfather always carried it in his pocket. And I know he had at least a hundred pounds in there, because he gave me some money out of it before we left home tonight."

Inspector Burk was still studying the room. On a table near where the body lay there was a liquor bottle, a beer bottle, and two glasses. There were also a number of cigarette butts. Some were in an ashtray, but one was on the sofa, two others on the floor close beside it. "Did your grandfather smoke cigarettes?" Burk asked.

"No sir. And neither my brother nor I smoke."

"Strange . . ." Burk said, half under his breath. But he was not referring to the fact that none of the Dinivans smoked. He had noticed that although the cigarettes looked as if they had been carelessly dropped where they lay, none of them had burned the area around it. So they must have been put out before they were dropped, he thought.

There was one other item that caught his attention. On the sofa, half-buried back of one of the pillows, was a woman's hair curler. Burk lifted it carefully with a handkerchief. "Is this yours?" he asked Hilda.

Her face reddened slightly. "No sir. I—I don't think I've ever seen one just like it before. It looks old-fashioned."

"So it does. Do you have any idea how it might have got here?"

It was Hilda's brother who answered. "Grandfather didn't expect us to get home early tonight. And—well, I know that sometimes he brought women here, prostitutes he picked up on the street."

To Inspector Burk that seemed, at first, to be the only lead he had. Certainly it was the obvious one: Walter Dinivan had received a woman visitor. Either he had opened his safe to give her money, or she already knew that he kept the key in his pocket. She had tried to strangle him, but not being strong enough, she then hit him over the head with some weapon that she later took away with her.

Even so, there were things about this story that troubled the inspector. His fingerprint experts had found only one print in the room that did not belong to Walter Dinivan or his grandchildren. This was a thumbprint on the beer glass. But would a person who had been so careless as to leave cigarette butts and a hair curler behind have managed to leave only one print?

Then there was the hair curler. Burk's detectives had questioned every known prostitute in the area. Several admitted knowing Walter Dinivan, but nobody recognized the hair curler. Instead they laughed at the idea of using such an old-fashioned article. And there was no evidence that one of them had seen Dinivan on the night of his death.

It occurred to Burk that Hilda and her brother might have murdered their grandfather, but the more he checked the less this seemed possible. They had gone to the dance, just as they told him. From the dance they had gone straight home and had phoned the police within minutes afterward.

The only clue left was the cigarettes that seemed to have been carelessly dropped, but no one of which had burned the rug or sofa beneath it. These were a popular brand smoked by thousands of persons.

From Hilda the inspector got a list of all Walter Dinivan's acquaintances and began to check them. Here he stumbled on information. One man who occasionally borrowed small sums from Dinivan was an old retired soldier named Joseph Williams. And it turned out that just one day after Dinivan's death, Williams had begun to pay off debts that he had owed for months.

Science Catches the Criminal

Inspector Burk went to call on Joseph Williams. He found an old man scrawny and weak of body but fiery of temperament. When Burk introduced himself, Williams let out a scream. "I know why you're here! You want to accuse me of killing old Dinny! Well, you're crazy, crazy!"

"I'm not trying to accuse you," Burk explained. "I'm trying to question the people who knew Mr. Dinivan. You did know him?"

"Know him? Of course I knew him!" Williams screamed. "I saw him the afternoon before he was killed. Met him on the street. He invited me in for a beer."

"How long were you there?"

"Long enough to drink one beer. Five minutes maybe. And it's none of your business!"

"Did he loan you money?"

"Two pounds. Not as much as I asked for." Suddenly the old man grabbed an ancient sword off the wall and began to wave it. "So that's what you're thinking!" he shouted. "You know that I got some money next day. Well, I won it at the races. Maybe I used old Dinny's money for the first bet, but the money I won belongs to me. Now get out of here!"

That was all Inspector Burk could get from Williams. Still, it made clear that the old man had a fierce temper and was somewhat mentally unbalanced. Also, if Walter Dinivan had taken the money he loaned Williams out of his safe, then Williams must have known about the safe and the key.

Inspector Burk went to call on Mrs. Williams, a rather plump old lady who had been separated from her husband for several years. Yes, she said, when the inspector showed her the hair curler, that was the kind she used. And yes, she might have left one behind when she moved out of Williams' house. But she couldn't be sure.

Burk began to feel certain that Williams was the killer. Surely he had known about Dinivan's custom of taking streetwalkers to his home. Then he could have planted the cigarettes and hair curler to make it look as if a woman was the murderer.

But how could this be proved? Even if the thumbprint on the beer glass turned out to be Williams', he could say it had been left in the afternoon.

The cigarettes were something else. Williams said he had been in the house only five minutes. In that time he could not have smoked the six cigarettes Burk had found. Also, Dinivan's granddaughter was certain the cigarette butts had not been there when she and her brother left to go dancing.

Inspector Burk sent the cigarette butts to a man named Roche Lynch.

Roche Lynch was a most unlikely looking detective. He was in his fifties, a tiny little man but a dapper dresser, always with a carnation in his buttonhole. His face was thin with puckered lines around his eyes from long hours of peering into a microscope. Roche Lynch was a medical detective, the most famous serologist—a specialist in blood serums—in all England.

Since Paul Uhlenhuth had learned how to tell the blood of one animal from that of another, other doctors had gained important new knowledge about the properties of blood. Even before Uhlenhuth's time doctors had occasionally, in grave emergencies, tried blood transfusions from one person to another. Now and then this was successful; in other cases the patient died, and no one understood why. This was the problem on which a Dr. Karl Landsteiner was working.

Landsteiner began using the blood of the other scientists in the laboratory where he worked. First, just as Uhlenhuth had done, he separated the serum—the liquid part of the blood—from the cells. Then he put the serum from a Dr. Stork's blood in six different test tubes. To each of these he added blood cells from one of the other doctors in the lab. In some of the tubes there was an instant agglutination. But in other tubes nothing happened at all.

Apparently the blood of some human beings was compatible with that of some other persons, but not with all. This would explain why a blood transfusion sometimes worked and sometimes failed. But what caused this difference in human blood?

Eventually Landsteiner decided that human blood contained two kinds of cell characteristics which he called A and B. However, the serum of some persons would, for some unknown reason, act against characteristic A, making its existence impossible. The serum of other persons would act against B. And there was still another group where the serum would act against both A and B. At first Landsteiner called this group C. Later other doctors joined with Landsteiner in his work, and it was learned that all human blood could be classified in four major types now called

A, B, O (which Landsteiner had originally called C), and AB. This last type is the rarest of all; it flows in the veins of only about 3 to 5 per cent of the people, and it contains the characteristics of both A and B.

The blood type of every human being could be determined by agglutination tests much like those Uhlenhuth had used to tell the blood of a pig from that of a horse.

Dr. Landsteiner would continue his experiments for the rest of his life, gaining new information. And one of these experiments must have surprised the doctor himself. He learned that blood was not the only thing which could be classified in the types A, B, AB, and O. In a large majority of people the bodily secretions such as sweat, saliva, and urine could be typed exactly like blood. And if a man's blood was type A, then so was his saliva. If his blood was type B, his sweat was type B. On the other hand there were a few persons whose secretions contained no characteristics and so could not be typed. Doctors called these "nonsecretors."

Inspector Burk had only recently read of this discovery. Now he sent the cigarettes found near Walter Dinivan's body to the one man he thought might be able to help him, Roche Lynch.

It did not take Lynch long to make his tests. Whoever had smoked these cigarettes was a secretor. And the saliva left on them clearly showed that the smoker belonged to Blood Group AB—the rarest of all groups.

Now the problem was back to Burk. Under British law he could not force Williams to have a blood test made. So what?

Burk and another detective began to follow Williams, keeping out of sight. When they saw him enter a bar, both men followed. Burk greeted Williams as if totally surprised to see him. "I'm sorry if I caused you any trouble the other day," he said. "Just doing my job, you know."

"Job!" Williams snarled. "Hounding innocent citizens!"

"Well, that's past. Let me buy you a drink."

Williams made a snorting noise, but he accepted the drink. He accepted the cigarette Burk offered. And later when he dropped it on the floor, Burk's friend quietly picked it up.

The cigarette butt went to Roche Lynch. Word came back that the smoker belonged to Blood Group AB. Williams was arrested and charged with the murder of Walter Dinivan.

At the trial it was shown that the thumbprint on the beer glass beside Dinivan's body had been made by Williams. But that, Williams said, was from the afternoon when he admitted visiting Dinivan. The hair curler was the kind Williams' wife used, but other persons used this kind also. The money Williams had spent after Dinivan's death might have been won at the racetrack.

Then there was the matter of the cigarettes and the tests made on them. Williams' attorney attempted to make a joke of the whole thing. British law had never heard of such a thing, he said. Certainly most of the jury had not. To many of them it sounded like a fairy tale—claiming a man could take a single cigarette smoked hours or even days before and from it tell the blood type of the smoker.

Joseph Williams was acquitted and turned free.

A newspaperman named Norman Rae offered to drive Williams to his home after the trial. He thought the reaction of the bitter, vindictive old man would make a good story.

It turned out to be a far better story than Rae had expected, but one he could not use for a number of years. Williams had asked to be taken to his old home town of Poole. "I want to see their faces when I walk up the street," he said. "They all thought I'd hang, damn them!"

It was a long drive and they stopped that night at a hotel near Dorchester. Williams began to drink. "To the hangman!" he cried, waving his glass. "To the hangman who's been cheated of his victim!" He took a long swallow. "To Inspector Burk and all his crazy cronies. May they rot in hell!"

Finally Rae got the old man to bed. Then he went to his own room next door.

Several hours later he was awakened by a pounding on the door. When he opened it, Williams staggered in. His eyes were wild, his mouth shaking. "I've got to tell somebody!" he whispered, "I've got to. I'll never sleep if I don't."

"Tell what?"

"That I killed Dinny. I killed him, just like they said. They couldn't prove it. But I did. And I had to tell somebody before I can sleep."

Still sobbing, the old man went back to his room. Next morning he appeared to have forgotten the whole thing. Rae drove him to the town of Poole, then returned to his newspaper.

Science Catches the Criminal

Under British law Williams could not be tried twice for the same crime. Once acquitted, he was free to brag about it, even to the police, if he wished. He was also free to claim that any story Rae published was false and then sue the newspaper for libel. So the reporter waited, and it was only after the death of Joseph Williams that he published the story of what had happened that night.

The Case of the Murdered Flea

Not every man suspected by the police is guilty. About the time Joseph Williams was being acquitted of the murder of Walter Dinivan in England, another murder was being investigated in Turin, Italy. One suspect was arrested largely because of stains on his trousers that appeared to be blood. The trousers were sent to Dr. Leone Lattes for tests.

Most of the stains, Dr. Lattes reported, were made by wine, not blood. But there was one bloodstain—inside one of the pockets. The suspect had no explanation for whose blood it was, or how it had gotten there.

Further tests showed the blood to be type A, the same as the victim's. It was also the same as the suspect's. It could be either.

Dr. Lattes put the bloodstained bit of pocket under the microscope. One look and he began to laugh. Crushed into the fibers of the cloth were the remains of a flea. Obviously the flea had filled itself with the suspect's blood, and then been crushed. "We cannot say this man is so gentle he would not kill a flea," Dr. Lattes reported. "But we have no evidence he has killed anything larger."

The Man Who Learned Too Much

Ed Finnerty, nightwatchman for a building on West 30th Street in New York, stood on the front step smoking. It was 2:30 in the morning of March 30, 1943. There was no traffic and in the quietness Finnerty heard the sound of a door closing. He glanced toward the old rooming house next door.

From where he stood Finnerty's view of the rooming house steps was partially blocked by a high bannister. Above this, in the darkness, he could barely make out the stooped figure of a man. The man was coming down the steps backward, apparently pulling something heavy after him.

Finnerty grinned knowingly. The rooming house was old, rundown, most of its tenants poor. Now and then one of them sneaked away at night, carrying his possessions with him but leaving his rent unpaid. Finnerty guessed that this was what was happening now. But when the stooped man reached the sidewalk he straightened up and walked off, leaving whatever he had been dragging behind him.

That was odd, Finnerty thought, but really none of his business. He puffed quietly on his pipe for a few minutes. And then, simply to kill time, he strolled down the sidewalk to the building next door.

Science Catches the Criminal

In the darkness he almost stumbled over the body of a woman. She half lay, half sat, propped against one corner of the steps. Her head was bent curiously to one side, her mouth open. "Hey!" Finnerty said. "What—?" There was no answer and he did not expect one. Even in the darkness he felt sure the woman was dead.

Finnerty hurried back to his own building, meaning to call the police. But as he reached his front door he heard steps coming along the sidewalk. Hidden in the shadows of his doorway, Finnerty waited.

A small man came down the walk. He looked like the same man who had hurried away a few minutes before, but Finnerty couldn't be sure. He went past the woman on the walk, apparently without seeing her, up the steps and into the building.

Finnerty was uncertain what to do. Should he rush inside and call the police? Should he watch to see if the man came out again? Was this the same man he'd seen dragging something down the steps? While he hesitated, the door of the rooming house opened once more and a man came out. Finnerty was sure this was the same man he'd seen entering only a few minutes before. The man carried a small package. Once more he passed the woman at the foot of the steps and walked away.

At this point a police patrol car came down the street. Finnerty hailed it, pointing excitedly toward the woman's body and toward the man who was a block away now, visible under a street light, walking steadily but not running. The police car speeded up, caught up with the walking man and brought him back to the rooming house.

He was small, middle-aged, and he spoke in a broken mixture of Greek and English difficult to understand. But gradually his story became clear. His name was John Manos. He worked as cook in a restaurant, lived in this rooming house. He did not know the dead woman, had never seen her before. It was true he had been in and out of the house several times that night. This was because he had been sick the day before; all day he had stayed in his room without going out, without food. Tonight he felt better and had gone out for food. When he came back he noticed an empty wine bottle in his room. He was a neat man; the only reason he hadn't thrown the bottle away earlier was because he had been sick. So he had gone out again to throw the bottle away. It was wrapped in newspaper because people in this rooming house were not supposed to drink.

But the dead woman? He repeated over and over that he had never seen her. She had never been in his room. In fact, no one ever came in his room. He kept it clean himself and not even the rooming house maid was allowed inside.

Detectives had reached the scene before Manos finished his story and he had to go all over it again. The dead woman had never been in his room. No one ever entered his room.

By their flashlights the detectives examined the scene. The dead woman was in her fifties; she wore a green dress and a cheap black-and-white coat. There was a silk stocking and high-heeled shoe on her right leg, but her left shoe was missing.

Science Catches the Criminal

The detectives went up to Manos' room. It was sparsely furnished, extremely clean. There was no sign the woman had ever been here, no sign of a struggle. The room next to Manos was occupied by an old man who said that he too had been sick the day before and had not gone out. Nor had he been able to sleep tonight. The walls between the rooms were so thin that almost any sound in one room was audible in the other. The old man had heard Manos go in and out, but there had been no other sound. No voices. No struggle. He was certain there had been no one in Manos' room that night.

Experts from the police laboratory arrived to search the room for blood. Fresh blood may be washed clean with scrubbing, but it is almost impossible to remove the signs of dried blood. Wood may be soaked in water for days on end and still show the signs of dried blood. Also, scientists had developed new means of discovering bloodstains even where they had been washed clean while fresh. Manos' room was examined by ultraviolet light under which old bloodstains will show black. So will certain other stains, but there was nothing suspicious here. The room was darkened and sprayed with luminol: touched by luminol, even old bloodstains take on a strange bluish-white luminescence.

There was no sign of blood in Manos' neat room. Nor were there any fingerprints except those of Manos himself.

By this time police had a preliminary report from the medical examiner. The woman had been strangled by a man's hands. The marks of the fingers were clear on her neck. The autopsy was not yet complete and the time of death uncertain.

70

The dead woman was identified as Alice Persico. She was divorced from her husband and lived with a brother only a few blocks from Manos' rooming house. Her brother told the police that Alice drank a lot. Sometimes she would be gone for several days at a time, and he had no idea where she had been on the night of her death. He did know that she had a lover named Coyle, a violent-tempered man of whom Alice was afraid.

Police located Coyle. He was sick in a hospital and unable to leave his bed.

The police found Alice Persico's former husband. He was living in Brooklyn and could prove he hadn't been in Manhattan.

That left John Manos. Finnerty, the nightwatchman, now felt sure Manos was the person he had seen dragging something heavy out of the rooming house. That something had to be the body of Alice Persico. Also, Manos admitted going past the body several times without stopping; he claimed he had never seen it, but this seemed almost impossible. Still, Finnerty could not swear Manos was the person he had seen. And all the police checking could turn up no other evidence against the little man. He swore over and over that no one even entered his room.

The police search did, however, discover another clue. In a garbage can several blocks from Manos' house they found Alice Persico's missing shoe and her hat. These were wrapped in a man's worn undershirt along with two soiled handkerchiefs. But neither the undershirt nor the handkerchiefs had any laundry mark that could be traced.

Manos was still being held by police. Two detectives took the undershirt and handkerchiefs to his room, planning to check them against his other clothing. It was night when they entered the room. While one detective fumbled for the light switch, the other turned on his flashlight. Its beam touched on a dully glowing spot on the linoleum floor near the bed. The spot had not been made by blood. Earlier tests had proved that. But what was it?

Detective John Hawthorne was not a scientist. But he knew something about the work being done in the New York Medical Examiner's office. So he cut the spot out of the linoleum and took it, along with Manos' undershirts and handkerchiefs, to Dr. Alexander S. Wiener.

Dr. Wiener was still a young man but already one of the most famous serologists in the world. He had studied under the great Karl Landsteiner, had helped in the development of the blood grouping tests, and of even newer discoveries. More than any other one man Dr. Wiener was responsible for the knowledge that body secretions other than blood could be classified. Now he began work with a test for John Manos' blood type. It was B. The blood of Alice Persico had already been typed—A.

Next Dr. Wiener went to work on the undershirt and the handkerchiefs. The undershirt was sweat-stained and whoever had worn it had been a secretor, type B. The handkerchiefs were soiled by both mucus and sweat, both type B. So they might have belonged to Manos. On the other hand, there were at least a million other persons in New York who were also type B, so this was no real proof.

Now Dr. Wiener began work on the small piece of linoleum cut from Manos' floor. His first tests showed it had been made by edema fluid, a liquid the human body produces to soothe damaged tissues. It nearly always occurs in the throat of anyone being strangled, and usually some of it will spill out of the victim's mouth. Edema fluid, like sweat or saliva, can be typed. Dr. Wiener's report read:

"In the grouping tests the extract [of the edema fluid] inhibited the anti-A serum but not the anti-B serum, proving that the secretion came from a Group A individual."

Here was proof that Manos had lied when he repeated, over and over, that no other person had ever entered his room. Also, the autopsy was now complete and police knew that Alice Persico had been dead for twelve hours or more when she was found. Therefore the fact that the old man in the room next to Manos had heard no struggle during the night did not prove her body was not already in the room.

The detectives working on the case felt certain Manos was the killer. But they were not at all sure this could be proved in court. Manos had only to change his story and say that a number of people had visited his room, any one of whom might have been Group A. A clever lawyer could destroy the nightwatchman's story that the man pulling something down the front steps of the rooming house had "looked like John Manos."

"What we really need is a confession," one of the detectives said.

There was no attempt to use force on the small, rather slow-witted man. Instead, a number of persons from the medical examiner's office began to visit him. Some of them spoke Greek and could talk with him easily. In a casual way they explained to him about blood types and how his own blood had been typed. They let him look through a microscope and see for himself how blood cells agglutinated when mixed with serum. They showed him how his own room had been searched with luminol and ultraviolet rays for bloodstains and none found. They explained to him how the pattern of spilled blood can tell a story of its own: if blood falls from a height of eight feet or more it breaks into tiny drips; if the blood falls only a few inches each drop stays round, but as the height increases each drop tends to become more star-shaped; if the blood source is in motion—a person walking, or blood splashed from a swinging knife or hammer—the drops are tear-shaped, and the tail of the tear points in the direction of the motion.

For six weeks the education of John Manos continued. He became quite an authority on the use of blood in criminal detection. Possibly he wondered what was the purpose of all this, since he knew perfectly well no blood had been spilled in his room. But the subject began to fascinate him.

And then, still casually, the detectives told him how other body secretions could be classified. Again they let him actually seen the agglutination of cells, this time in sweat and saliva. They showed him the undershirt that had been wrapped around Alice Persico's missing shoe. They let him see that the sweat staining it was the same type as his own.

Then they let him see the edema-stained bit of linoleum cut from his floor and explained this was Group A, Alice Persico's.

Manos' face had a dazed look. He shook his head. "I did not think I would be caught," he said. "I did not understand."

In his broken English he explained then what had happened. He had gone out at night for a bottle of wine, and on the way back to his room met Alice Persico. He did not know her, but she spoke to him. He asked if she wanted some wine, and she went to his room with him. It turned out she was already drunk. A few more drinks and she became noisy. He was, as he had told the police, a quiet, neat man. He was afraid if she made a disturbance he would be put out of the rooming house. He had tried to make her be quiet, his hand over her mouth. She struggled; he hadn't really meant to choke her . . .

When he realized she was dead, he didn't know what to do. For a long time he sat and looked at the body. Then it was daylight and he could not move her. But he did not go to work. He stayed in his room and carefully cleaned everything, removing all fingerprints. When it was night again he waited until after two o'clock, then carried her body downstairs and out the door. He went back and found that her hat and shoe had been left behind. He wrapped these in an old undershirt—why he had included the handkerchiefs he could not remember—and took them away. He had just got rid of them when the police stopped him.

"I knew there were no fingerprints," he said. "No blood. Who would have thought that one little drop of water out of her mouth would make a difference."

The Future of Blood Tests—and The Case of the Unlikely Twins

Ralf and Irene Schnug were giving a party at their home in Basel, Switzerland. It was a large party; some of the guests were friends of friends whom the Schnugs knew only slightly, but everything was going happily. About eight o'clock Willi, the Schnug's five-year-old son, came in to say good night.

Konrad and Marie Mueller were on the far side of the room when Willi entered. Konrad did not see the child at first, but Marie did. She caught her breath so sharply that Konrad asked, "What happened?"

Before she could answer Irene Schnug came across the room, leading the child. "This is my son Willi," she said to the Muellers.

Now both the Muellers were staring at the child. "Willi?" Mrs. Mueller said, her voice barely audible. Then she laughed, shaking her head. "He looks so much like our son Hans that for a moment . . . It's amazing."

"Amazing!" her husband repeated. "From across the room I would have sworn it was Hans. How old is he?"

"Five."

"The same as Hans," Mrs. Mueller said.

At this point someone else joined the group, laughing and bringing drinks. Nothing else was said about the child. But neither Mr. nor Mrs. Mueller could stop thinking about the extraordinary resemblance between Willi and their son Hans. When they reached home they immediately went to their children's bedroom.

They had twin sons, Hans and Eric. The two boys lay side by side asleep. They did not look at all like one another. But the resemblance between Hans and Willi Schnug was incredible.

Staring at the sleeping children Mrs. Mueller said, "I wonder where Willi was born, and what day . . ."

Her husband understood what she meant. "That's impossible. Hospitals never mix children. Anyway, Willi probably was born somewhere else."

"But I've got to know," Mrs. Mueller said.

She went to the telephone and called Irene Schnug. She apologized for calling at such a late hour. "But I had to ask. What is your son Willi's birthday?"

"February 6."

Mrs. Mueller gasped. "The same as Hans and Eric! And where—?"

"In Hospital Gnade, here in Basel. Where were your twins born?"

"The same place."

The next day the two families got together, and now it was the Schnugs' turn to stare in surprise. Standing side by side, Hans Mueller and Willi Schnug looked like doubles. Eric, the same age and size, looked like neither. Together the families visited the Hospital Gnade. There the administrator swore it was impossible for the babies to have been mixed. "Blood tests will prove it," he said.

A child's blood type is inherited from its parents. If two parents both have Group A blood, their child cannot have Group B; if both parents have Group B their child cannot have A. So it is sometimes possible to tell that a certain person could *not* be the parent of a certain child. On the other hand, it is impossible to tell that any one person *is* the parent.

When the Muellers and Schnugs were tested, it turned

out that all four parents and all three children had Group A blood. So any one of the children *might* have been the child of any of the four parents.

The doctor who had made the tests came to Mr. Mueller. "I'm not a specialist in this field," he said. "I can work only with the basic blood groups, the A, B, AB, and O, that have been known for a long time now. But there is a doctor in New York City you should contact. His name is Alexander Wiener."

Scientists around the world had been carrying on the work begun years before by Paul Uhlenhuth and Karl Landsteiner. Of these, Alexander Wiener, who had helped solve the murder of Alice Persico, was probably the most famous. In his laboratory he had proved that the unique qualities of blood were not limited to the four basic groups Landsteiner had discovered. The strength of the A quality, for instance, could be divided into subgroups A1, A2, A3. Also, other major groups were discovered that came to be called M, N, and MN. Trying to find why some babies— called blue babies—were born with a mysterious ailment that often killed them in infancy, Dr. Wiener discovered a factor of blood that he called Rh positive and Rh negative. Indeed, by the 1970's Dr. Wiener and other scientists knew there were as many as fifteen major blood groups and five hundred or more subgroups. Since all these are inherited, it was possible to be much more exclusive about who *might* and *might not* be the parent of a certain child.

Dr. Wiener was fascinated by the problem of the Muellers and Schnugs. He asked that they send him a sample of blood from all seven persons involved.

His tests were written down as:

Hans Mueller A1, MNRh1, Rh2

Eric Mueller A1, MNrh

Willi Schnug A1, MNRh1, Rh2 (exactly the same as
   Hans Mueller)

Marie Mueller A1, NRh1, Rh1

Irene Schnug A1, MNRh1, rh

Working all this out on a chart, Dr. Wiener found that Hans and Eric Mueller could *not* be brothers, but Hans and Willi *could* be brothers. Also, Eric could *not* be the child of Marie Mueller, but he *could* be the child of Irene Schnug.

By this time a number of famous European doctors had become interested in the case. More tests showed that both Hans Mueller and Willi Schnug were colorblind, but Eric was not. Also, a skin graft from Eric's body would be rejected by both Hans and Willi, but Hans and Willi would accept skin from each other.

There could no longer be any doubt. The hospital had somehow gotten the newborn babies mixed up. And so Willi Schnug became Willi Mueller, and Eric Mueller became Eric Schnug, and the Mueller and Schnug families became firm friends with everybody feeling somehow kin to everybody else.

All over the world scientists continue to work on the mysteries of human blood and almost every year brings new discoveries. At the same time, almost every discovery opens the door to new mysteries beyond. Many scientists now believe that eventually it will be possible to identify every individual by his blood. Then, if a murderer or a thief left one drop of his blood behind, it would be like leaving a clearly etched fingerprint.

5

THE CROSSWORD PUZZLES
OF CRIME

Voice of the Dead

At 6:48 on the morning of May 7, 1964, the control
tower at the Oakland, California, airport had a call from
Pacific Airlines Flight 773. It was a routine call; Flight
773 came in every morning from Reno, Nevada, loaded
chiefly with persons who had been gambling all night and
now were taking the early flight back to work. The control
tower operator recognized the voice of Copilot Raymond
Andress giving his position as forty miles east, due to touch
down in sixteen minutes.

The tower operator spotted the flight on his radar, then
gave the usual weather data. "Wind south southeast twelve
knots, light overcast at 1,600 feet, visibility ten miles."

Andress acknowledged the information, asked permission
to descend to 5,000 feet. The tower agreed. It was all a
very routine conversation.

United Airlines Flight 593 came on the air to give its
position. The Oakland tower warned it of the Pacific flight

a few miles north. The United flight answered that the plane was visible from the starboard window.

At this point the control tower received a message the operator could not understand. It was a jumble of sounds: a metallic banging, engine noises, blurred words. The operator waited for a repeat and after a moment heard a kind of cry, "uh—uh-uh . . ." That was all.

Looking down, he saw that Pacific Airlines Flight 773 had disappeared from the radar screen.

Hurriedly the tower called the United Airlines Flight 593. "Is the Pacific plane still visible to your starboard?"

There was a pause. "Negative. Negative." And then suddenly, "There's a column of smoke coming up from the ground! I don't know what from. It wasn't there a moment ago!"

Some thirty-five miles east of the Oakland tower a rancher was watching his cattle, not from horseback but standing beside a pickup truck. It was not yet seven o'clock in the morning; the sun was still hidden beyond the rolling hills, but its upslanting light made the sky a clear blue and silver. It glittered on the wings of the Fairchild F-27. From below the rancher watched it idly. He knew that it passed over every morning at this hour.

Abruptly the plane nosed forward. It swerved to one side, back again. The nose went down more steeply, straight down, the engines running full throttle. The rancher could only watch, unmoving, mouth open.

The earth shook with the impact. A tremendous ball of red-and-orange flame, laced with smoke, shot skyward.

Without knowing he had moved, the rancher jumped into his truck and headed for the nearest telephone.

The first persons to reach the scene were deputies from the Contra Costa County sheriff's office and members of the California Highway Patrol. They stood and stared in awe. The plane had struck the ground intact, but the wreckage had been hurled hundreds of feet in every direction. And scattered with the wreckage of the plane were bits of human bodies. One of the officers turned away and was sick.

Close on the heels of the officers came the curious and souvenir seekers—those strange people who, with the instinct of buzzards, are automatically drawn to the scene of a tragedy. They come not to help but to stare, to feed themselves on the sight of death. The police roped off the entire area to hold these people back. They began the gruesome task of gathering the shattered bits of what had been human bodies.

Next—and with amazing speed, since some of them had to come from as far away as Washington—were the scientific detectives. There were ten men from the CAB, the Civil Aeronautics Board. They were former pilots, aviation engineers, men who knew the structure of an airplane from its nose to its tail. With them were other engineers from Fairchild, the plane's manufacturer, from Rolls Royce which had made the engines, and from the company that made the propellers.

Together these men studied the scene and photographed it in detail. Bit by bit they began to pick up the wreckage. The exact spot where each piece was found was marked on a chart. And the wreckage itself, little by little, was put together in a mock-up of the plane.

Where there was any question in the scientists' minds, the pieces of the plane were analyzed by spectrograph. This is an instrument that can transform energy into visible form. When any substance is heated, its atomic arrangement is disturbed. The disturbed atoms send off energy waves composed of different colors. The spectrograph can chart these and so pinpoint the most minute amount of any substance present. If the plane had been blown up in mid-air by dynamite or any other explosive, the spectrograph would find traces of it.

But Flight 773 had not been blown up. It had been intact, the engines functioning perfectly, when it hit the ground. The engines themselves were buried so deeply a power shovel had to be used to uncover them.

It was at this time that one of the deputy sheriffs found a Smith and Wesson .357 magnum revolver, a gun so powerful it could send a bullet through the engine block of an automobile. At first it was thought to belong to an off-duty policeman who had been on the plane; but then it was learned that the policeman had owned no such gun.

Analysis showed that the gun had been loaded with six bullets and all had been fired recently. But exactly how recently it was impossible to say.

All this time a different group of scientific detectives were at work trying to make sense of the garbled radio message which had been received by the Oakland control tower. The message had, like all others, been automatically taped. But simply playing it back, listening with the human ear, was no help. It still remained an unintelligible jumble of sound.

So, for the first time in the solution of a major crime, an invention called a "sound spectrogram" came into use.

The human voice is "shaped" by the throat, mouth, nasal passages, along with the lips, teeth, tongue, and other organs. All these differ somewhat from one person to another, and some acoustical engineers have long believed that the voice would prove as individual as fingerprints—if there was just some way to catch and show this difference.

During World War II, U.S. Naval scientists began studying the voices of Japanese radio operators: if the voice of one operator could be absolutely identified, then the unit to which he was attached might be traced. After the war, Bell Telephone scientists continued these studies. If one voice could be separated from all others, then a tape might be made of, say, ten persons talking at the same time; by separating one voice at a time from all the others, then each speech would become distinct.

In their experiments the scientists again made use of the spectrograph's ability to change energy into visible form. Using a vastly complicated machine, the energy used in speaking could be transformed into jagged lines on a sheet of paper. To most persons these lines would have less meaning than a baby's scribbling. To the expert they represented not only words, but words formed by a specific human voice.

This was the gadget used to unscramble the message received by the Oakland tower.

First, filters of one kind and another were used to take

out all unnecessary sounds. The blurred words that remained were compared with other tapes of Copilot Raymond Andress' voice. It was determined that Andress had sent the message, but his words were still unintelligible.

The scientists made a sound spectrogram of the entire message. From this some of the words could be read. Against the shape of the others, the scientists tested one word after another in their own voices. Finally it read: "Skipper's shot. We've been shot. (I was) trying to help." The words "I was" were put in parentheses because the men studying the voice print could never be absolutely sure of them.

After this message there was a pause of several seconds. Then came brief sounds that were not words at all but gasping, a kind of "Uh . . . Uh . . ." And that was all.

It was enough to show that, somehow, the pilot and copilot of Flight 773 had been murdered.

The engineers putting together the wreckage of the plane soon verified this. A twisted piece of metal was identified as the back of the pilot's seat. Through this were two bullet holes.

Now the tracing of the pistol found in the wreck became vital. This was straight police work and comparatively easy. The pistol had been bought, just one day before the tragedy, by a man named Frank Gonzalez. Asking questions, the police learned that Gonzalez had been deeply in debt. Also he had been having family troubles. After buying the pistol he had borrowed several hundred dollars, then bought a round-trip ticket to Reno, Nevada. There he had gambled desperately, and lost. With his last few coins he

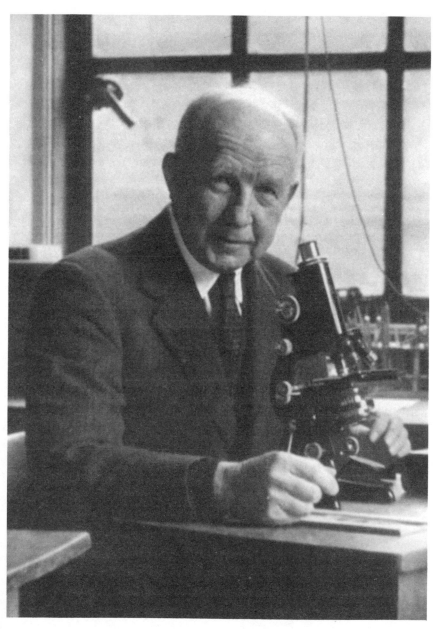

1. Sir Sydney Smith in his laboratory.

History of the
"West Brothers" Identification..

Bertillon Measurements are not always a Reliable Means of Identification

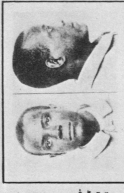

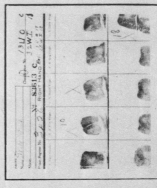

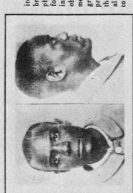

In 1903, one WILL WEST was committed to the U. S. Penitentiary at Leavenworth, Kansas, a few days thereafter being brought to the office of the record clerk to be measured and photographed. He denied having been in the penitentiary before, but the clerk doubting the statement, ran his measuring instruments over him, and from the Bertillon measurements obtained went to his files, returning with the card the measurements called for properly filled out, accompanied with the photograph and bearing the name WILLIAM WEST. Will West, the new prisoner, continued to deny that the card was his, whereupon the record clerk turned it over and read that William West was already a prisoner in that institution, having been committed to a life sentence on September 9, 1901, for murder.

The Bertillon measurements of these, given below, are nearly identical whereas the fingerprint classifications given are decidedly different.

The case is particularly interesting as indicating the fallacies in the Bertillon system, which necessitated the adoption of the fingerprint system as a medium of identification. It is not even definitely known that these two Wests were related despite their remarkable resemblance.

Their Bertillon measurements and fingerprint classifications are set out separately below:

177.5; 188.0; 91.3; 19.8; 15.9; 14.8; 6.5; 27.5; 12.2; 9.6; 50.3
15- 30 W OM 13 :Ref: 30 W OM 13
28 W I   26 U OO

178.5; 187.0; 91.2; 19.7; 15.8; 14.8; 6.6, 28.2; 12.3; 9.7; 50.2
10- 13 U O O Ref: 13 U O 17
32 W I 18   28 W I 18

2. The Bertillon measurements are not always reliable, as shown here

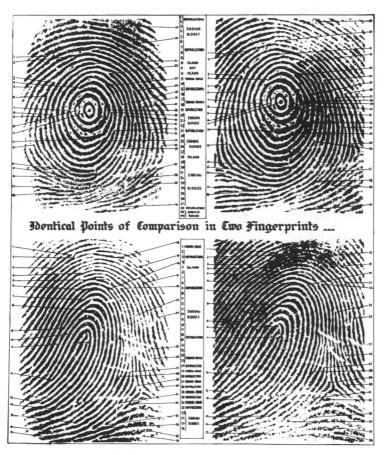

3. *Fingerprint comparison.*

Mother Finds Son Lost to Her for 17 Years.
Another Instance Proving That ...

Fingerprints Never Change

ON AUGUST 10, 1944, the Federal Bureau of Investigation, United States Department of Justice, Washington, D. C., received a request from a mother at Yakima, Washington, for assistance in locating her son whom she had not seen in 17 years. When the son was four years old, his father had placed him in a home to be adopted. The father had been dead 13 years, and the mother's efforts to find her son were of no avail until she sought the assistance of the FBI.

Accompanying her request was a set of fingerprints taken when the boy was three years old. When checked in the FBI Identification Division, they were found to be identical with those of a young man who had enlisted in the United States Navy at Des Moines, Iowa, in 1941. After 15 years, his fingerprints were unchanged, and the mother at last learned her son's whereabouts.

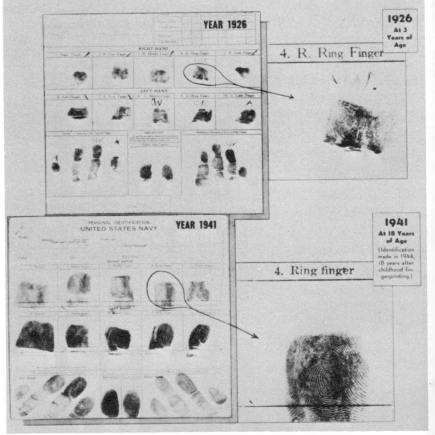

4. Fingerprints remain the same throughout a person's lifetime.

5. *Identification from a fingertip removed by a bite.*

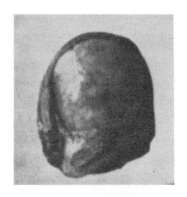

(Right) Tip of finger with nail.

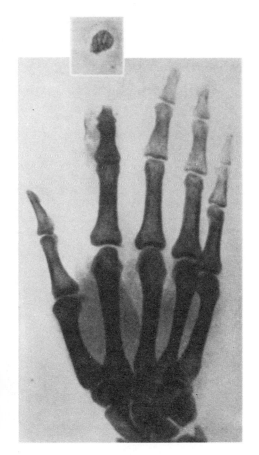

(Above) Right index finger of accused.

(Left) X-ray of accused's right hand. This shows the fracture of the end of the index finger. Inset is an X-ray of the fingertip.

FEDERAL BUREAU OF INVESTIGATION
UNITED STATES DEPARTMENT OF JUSTICE

ROSCOE PITTS

MUTILATION OF FINGERPRINTS

This case accents the futility of attempting to alter or destroy fingerprints

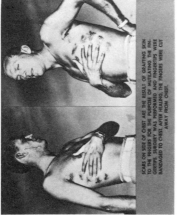

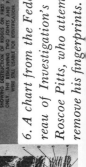

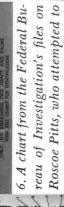

CLOSE-UP OF TWO OF THE MUTILATED FINGERTIPS CLEARLY SHOWS THAT RIDGE ON SECOND JOINT WERE UNCHANGED.

SCARS ON SIDE OF CHEST ARE THE RESULT OF GRAFTING SKIN TO THE FINGERS FOR THE PURPOSE OF MUTILATING THE FINGERTIPS. SURGERY WAS PERFORMED AND FINGERTIPS WERE BANDAGED TO CHEST. AFTER HEALING, THE FINGERS WERE CUT AWAY FROM CHEST.

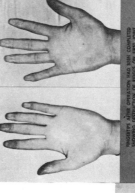

FINGERTIPS AFTER OPERATION HAD BEEN COMPLETED SHOWING DESTRUCTION OF RIDGES ON FIRST JOINT ONLY. THE REMAINING TWO JOINTS AND PALMS WERE STILL USABLE FOR IDENTIFICATION.

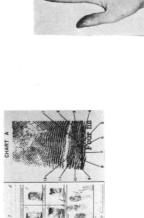

6. A chart from the Federal Bureau of Investigation's files on Roscoe Pitts, who attempted to remove his fingerprints.

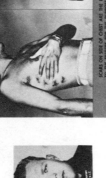

CHART A

CHART B

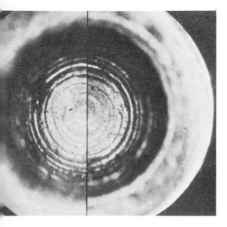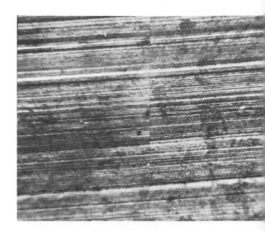

7. Left: *A photomicrograph of the firing pin indentations in the primers of two cartridge cases fired in the same gun.* 8. Right: *Comparison of two bullets by means of a photomicrograph.*

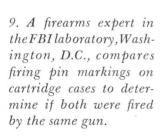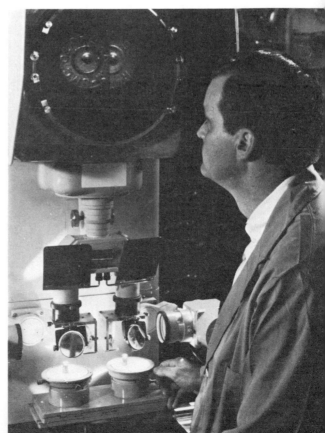

9. *A firearms expert in the FBI laboratory, Washington, D.C., compares firing pin markings on cartridge cases to determine if both were fired by the same gun.*

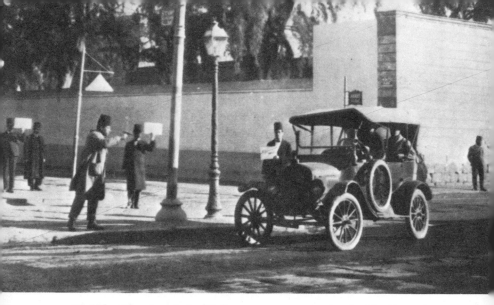

10. *The Murder of the Sirdar—a reconstruction by the Egyptian police of the crime.*

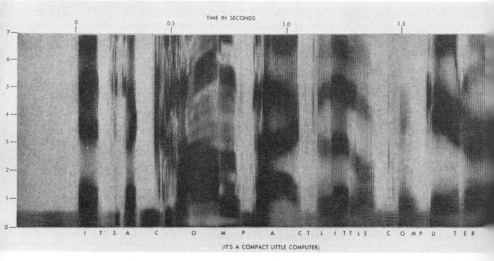

11. *An example of a sound spectrogram.*

INTERESTING SPEECH PATTERNS

WE   YOU

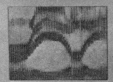 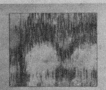

REALLY   REALLY (WHISPERED)

NUMBERS FREQUENTLY CONFUSED

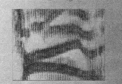 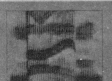 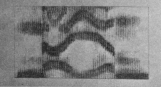

FIVE   NINE   NIYAN

WORDS THAT SOUND ALIKE LOOK ALIKE

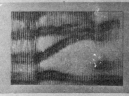 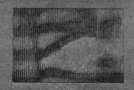 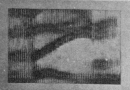

VEIN   VANE   VAIN

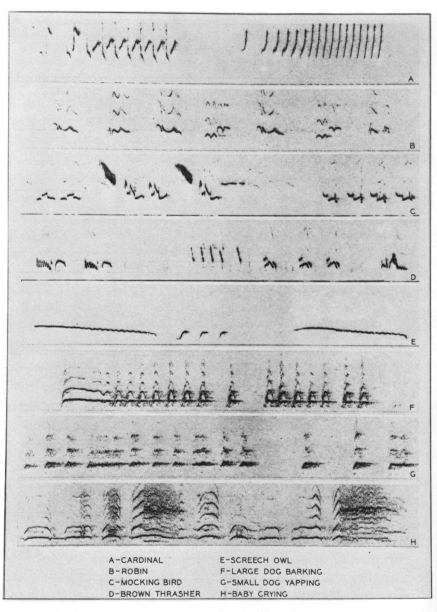

A–CARDINAL E–SCREECH OWL
B–ROBIN   F–LARGE DOG BARKING
C–MOCKING BIRD G–SMALL DOG YAPPING
D–BROWN THRASHER H–BABY CRYING

13. Comparison of various voices by sound spectrograms.

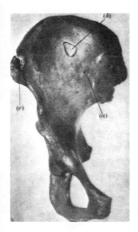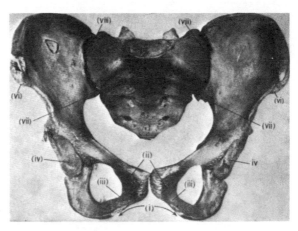

14. *The three bones taken from a well in Egypt. Left: The right hipbone,
(a) irregularly shaped lead slug embedded in the bone; (b) triangular
piece of bone, displaced by a slug; (c) grooved fracture, showing erosion
of bone due to septic infection after the passage of a slug.*

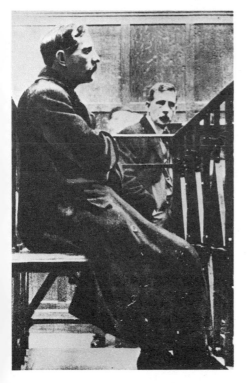

15. *George Joseph Smith*

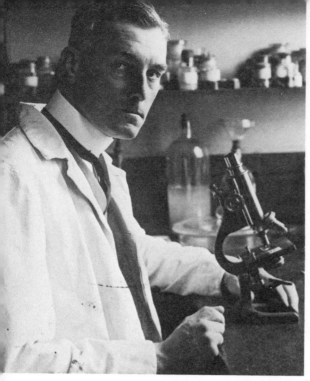

16. Sir Bernard Spilsbury in his laboratory

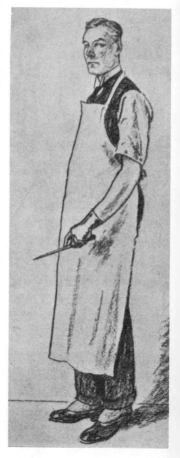

17. A cartoon of Sir Bernard Spilsbury

had bought airflight insurance and mailed this to his family. Then, in the cold, predawn darkness, he had gone aboard Flight 773.

Exactly what happened after that, no living person could ever be absolutely sure. But to the men studying the jagged lines of the sound spectrogram or looking at the bullet-pierced back of the pilot's seat it seemed fairly certain.

As the plane began to descend for its Oakland approach, Frank Gonzalez had finally carried out the plan that he must have made the day before. He was not thinking of the pilot, the copilot, or the other passengers as fellow human beings. He was thinking of his own troubles and of the the insurance that would pay off only if he died in a plane crash. He got out of his seat, pushed open the door to the cockpit, and began to shoot.

In the same month that California scientists were using the sound spectrogram to unravel the mystery of Flight 773, scientists on the opposite side of the United States were using it to solve an entirely different kind of crime.

One lovely May morning the telephone in the office of the Pitney Bowes manufacturing plant in Stamford, Connecticut, rang sharply. To the secretary who answered a man's voice, obviously disguised, said, "A bomb has been hidden in your plant. It's big enough to destroy the plant and everybody in it. Get everybody out, quick. This is your only warning." After that the phone went dead.

Immediately all the employees were dismissed and sent home. Experts were called in. Carefully, inch by inch, they searched for the bomb, never knowing when they might be blown up. Men who worked on the night shift were told not to come to work while the search went on.

No bomb was ever found.

Two weeks later there was a second bomb threat. Again, all the employees for the day and night shift were dismissed. And again no bomb was found.

Three days later came the third threat. For the third time all employees were sent home. And for the third time no bomb was found.

After the first call the police had suspected the whole thing was a hoax. Secretly they installed a machine to record any calls made to the plant office. So they had on tape the last two bomb threats.

A sound spectrogram was made of these calls. Already plant officials were listing a number of possible suspects. These were brought into the office on one pretext or another, and their voices secretly recorded, and made into spectrograms. These were compared to the voice of the pretended bomber.

The fact that the man making the threats had deliberately disguised his voice made no difference to the spectrogram. There was no way he could change the "shape" the spectrogram recorded. An expert studying the wiggled lines put his finger on one. "There's your man."

Confronted with this evidence, the man blushed a deep red. "Of course I wasn't going to use a real bomb," he said. "But the weather's been so pretty, I just wanted a few days off to go fishing."

The Crossword Puzzles of Crime

The Case of Three Bones

Bits and pieces of the human voice are not, of course, the only fragments from which the scientific detectives put together their crossword puzzles of crime. Take, for instance, the case of Dr. Sydney Smith—the same Dr. Smith who had matched the fingerprints from a piece of skin with what was left of a human hand—and his three small bones.

Police brought the bones to Dr. Smith's laboratory in Cairo, Egypt. "They were found in a well," he was told. "The well had been abandoned for a long time. Now it is about to be put in use again; so it was being cleaned, and these were found. We don't know if they are animal bones, or human, or what."

Next day Dr. Smith gave the police a written report. The bones, he said, were those of a young woman, probably between twenty-three and twenty-five years of age. She had been small and slender. Her left leg was slightly shorter than her right, so that she walked with a limp—possibly the result of polio as a child. She had borne at least one child. She had been killed, probably about three months earlier, by a shotgun loaded with homemade slugs. It had been fired from a position slightly lower than the girl's body, at close range, and the killer had been a little bit to the left. Also, she had not died immediately but several days later due to an infection following the shooting.

The police official who read the report shook his head. He had seen the bones—just three small bones with a tiny bit of rotten flesh clinging to one of them. Nobody, he thought, could look at three small bones and tell all this about them. The policeman went to call on Dr. Smith.

Smith spread the bones on his laboratory table. "These two," he said, "are hipbones." He placed the third bone between them so that they formed a rough triangle. "This is the sacrum. And together they make a pelvis. You can tell by the shape that it is that of a woman—the male pelvis is narrower. Also, these bones are light and small. They might almost be those of a child. But notice the crest of the hipbone." He touched it with a finger. "Here it becomes united when a person is somewhere between the age of twenty-two to twenty-five. Notice that this is almost united, but not quite. So she had to be in her early twenties."

The policeman nodded. "Go ahead."

"There was a fragment of flesh clinging to one bone when they were brought. In this hot climate bodies decay rapidly. I do not know the temperature in that well. So it's only a rough guess when I say she had been dead about three months. I could be a month or so off on that. And these grooves in the bones here show she'd had at least one child, maybe more. I can't tell."

"You said her right leg was longer than her left and she limped."

"Yes. Notice that the right hipbone is bigger and heavier than the left. Also the cavity in this hip where the head of the femur—the long leg bone—fits is bigger than in the left hip. That means the right hip has carried most of the body weight for a long time, probably since childhood. It's only a guess that this was because of polio."

"And the way she was killed?"

"There was a lead bullet in her right hip, but it was a crudely shaped, handmade bullet. And here—" he traced it with his finger —"this groove was made by another. Here another. That means it was a shotgun, fired at close range or the pellets would have been more widely spread. The slant of the grooves show the direction from which the gun was fired. Now if you'll study the edge of this groove with a magnifying glass you'll see that the bone has eroded, the result of infection. So she didn't die immediately after the shot."

The policeman went away shaking his head and still not quite convinced that Dr. Smith's magic was possible. But when he went to the neighborhood where the bones had been found and started to inquire about a young, crippled girl who had disappeared three or four months earlier he was told immediately, "You must mean the daughter of Ahmed Amer."

Amer was a poor man, uneducated. When the police began to question him he quickly confessed. "I didn't mean to kill her. I was cleaning my shotgun and she was standing in front of me when it went off. I was afraid to send for a doctor: I had no license for the gun and I knew I would be arrested if I explained what had happened. But I thought she was going to get well. Then—she died."

In terror of being arrested for murder, Amer had dropped his daughter's body in the well. It was an old well and had not been used for years. He did not think it ever would be used again. But when he heard that the well was to be reopened, he climbed down into it at night.

Science Catches the Criminal

By this time his daughter's body had almost completely decayed. He took away all he could and threw the bits into the Nile. But working in the darkness he had overlooked the three bones.

There was no real proof that Amer's story was true. Yet it matched exactly the points that Dr. Smith had made. Amer's neighbors all said he had truly loved his daughter. He was fined for owning an unlicensed gun and released.

The Eight Coats of Paint

The child was five years old. He had, apparently, slipped out of his house, planning to visit a friend a half block away. It was raining, hard. In the thickening twilight the headlights of autos showed only as misty blurs. When the child's mother missed him, she went to the door, expecting to find him on the porch, but he was not there.

She went back into the house, calling him. She couldn't believe he had gone outside in this weather. Eventually she called the home of his friend down the block. No, her son was not there. He hadn't been there that afternoon.

The mother was frantic now. The child's father came home. They went outside, in the pouring rain. The father walked one way, the mother the other. It was dark now and she passed the little bundle of torn clothing that lay in the gutter without seeing it. But on the way back toward her home, a half hour later, she walked close to the curb. And so she found her son's body. He had been killed by a hit-and-run driver as he started to cross the street.

The Crossword Puzzles of Crime

No one had seen the accident. The body had lain for more than an hour in the rain and mud. There seemed to be little chance of ever finding the killer.

This was in Seattle, Washington, in 1954, and the Seattle police laboratory was not equipped for the job that faced it. The child's clothing was sent to the F.B.I. laboratory in Washington, D.C.

There the technicians began a minute examination, piece by piece, of the clothing. Some was stained with blood, but the blood was that of the child. The mud was analyzed, and had come from the gutter in which the body lay. There were also several tiny fragments of paint.

The F.B.I. laboratory contains a national automobile paint file. Here are samples of every original finish put on automobiles in the United States. There are also samples of practically every other paint manufactured.

A scientist mounted one of the paint chips in plastic, then sliced through it with a sharp blade. Turned on edge and examined under a microscope, it was clear that the chip was composed of eight different coats of paint. One by one these eight layers were examined under a spectrograph. It worked on the principle that, heated, every element gave off energy in color that could be scientifically measured. So exact, so precise, was the spectrograph that the operator could tell what elements composed each layer of paint, and in what proportion. Each could then be checked against the laboratory's file of manufactured paints.

The eighth coat of paint—the newest one—on the chip being studied, was purple. It was not a type of paint used by an auto company as original finish. It was, however, a fairly common brand of paint that could be bought in many stores.

The coat beneath it was a black primer, obviously used to prepare for the purple finish. But it was the original coats that were of most importance. Studying these, comparing them with his file, the scientist was able to say definitely that this paint had been used exclusively on 1946-model Cadillacs.

So the car which had killed the child was a 1946 Cadillac, original color white, painted purple at the time of the accident.

There were not so many purple 1946 Cadillacs in Seattle that it took the police long to locate the one involved. The owner admitted having hit something the night the child was killed, but insisted he thought it was a dog. He had not stopped, he said, because of the pouring rain and because he thought there was nothing he could do.

The judge had no way of knowing if the man told the truth. The sentence he handed down was an odd one. The driver was sentenced to one year's probation. In that time he could not drive a car. He was also fined $1,000—and the money went into a police fund to reward informers in hit-and-run cases.

Science is sometimes used to solve mysteries less serious than a hit-and-run killing. Take what might be called The Case of the Boarding House Hash.

In this case the detective was a young medical student living in a Baltimore boarding house. He began to suspect that his landlady scraped off the food left each night on the dinner plates and used it again the next morning in hash. But how could he prove it?

One night the student left a scrap of beef on his plate and sprinkled on it a few grains of lithium chloride, a substance that looks and tastes like common salt. Next morning there was nothing about the hash that seemed different from usual, but the student wrapped a bit of it in paper and took it to the university laboratory. There he heated it over a Bunsen burner, then examined it under a spectroscope—and found a thin crimson line that proved the presence of lithium.

So the crime was solved, but the solution proved of little help to the young detective. As he later told a friend, "That boarding house was the cheapest one around. It was the only place I could afford to eat. I knew that if I complained to the landlady she'd throw me out. So I just kept on eating leftovers."

6

FIRES AND STRANGE FUELS

How and When Did He Die?

Approximately seven miles west of Massillon, Ohio, the tracks of the Pennsylvania Railroad are crossed by a small country road. This is a desolate, hilly area and the small road, where it crosses the tracks, is on a steep grade.

At 2:20 A.M. April 23, 1963, Pennsylvania train #50 was racing westward. Its headlight bored a tunnel through the darkness, glinting most of the time on steel tracks ahead, then sweeping across the countryside as the train rounded a curve. The engineer stood beside the cab window, relaxed. It was a run he had made many times before.

Suddenly a tremendous ball of flame leaped at him—or up from under him. He could never be sure. In that instant, half-blinded, he saw what seemed to be an automobile wrapped in flames and at the same time heard the grinding crash of it striking the train.

Instinctively the engineer brought the train to a halt. The fireman was saying repeatedly, "What happened? What was that?"

"I don't know." The engineer had the dazed impression

that it might have been a meteor, a comet. As the train came to a halt both he and the fireman jumped to the ground and went racing back down the tracks.

Fifty feet from a mass of flaming wreckage they stopped. The heat was too great for them to go closer. But they could tell it was an automobile, the gasoline tank exploded, wrapped in a mass of flame.

The fireman said in a whisper, "My God! I think there's a man in there!" He couldn't be sure. The heat burned his eyes and there was nothing he could do.

The engineer ran back to his cab to radio ahead what had happened. It was approximately twenty-nine minutes after the accident when the first law enforcement officers arrived. The wrecked car still burned, though the great mass of flame was gone. Another two hours or more would pass before the remains of what had once been a human body could be removed from the front seat. This was wrapped in a plastic sheet and carried to the nearest funeral home. From here it was taken to the Cuyahoga County coroner's office in Cleveland. Here Dr. Lester Adelson, Chief Deputy Coroner and Pathologist for Cuyahoga County, began his autopsy.

The autopsy began approximately twelve hours after train and auto smashed together. Later, a man's life would depend on this matter of time.

Even before the body could be removed from the automobile, police were picking through the wreckage scattered along the railroad tracks. They found credit cards, some burned to ash but others with the name Robert K. Domer still legible. There was a badly charred wallet with the name Robert Domer on it. And when police checked the license plate on the car they found it had been registered to Robert K. Domer of Canton, Ohio.

When police went to Domer's home, Mrs. Domer told them her husband had disappeared slightly more than three weeks before. Tearfully she gave them what might—or might not—be considered a strange kind of suicide note.

This was a tape recording. In it Domer did not actually speak of suicide, but of a separation from his wife. In one part he said, "If I don't do what I am about to do, I'm going to be separated from you anyway because you know very well when the circumstances and facts are known, this will be the only result possible."

At this point—it was still April 23, the day of what appeared to be Domer's death—the police set out to ask a lot more quesions about him. The answers came quickly—Robert Domer had been in deep trouble with the law.

Domer had been a huge man, weighing close to three hundred pounds, with a huge ambition to make a lot of money in a big hurry. He had owned a mortgage and loan company which, at first anyway, appeared to be tremendously successful. In January of that year it was supposed to have assets of $93 million. But when federal investigators began a routine check they found a number of things that required explanation. The investigators had kept checking—and on March 30 they informed Domer they had evidence he had stolen approximately $87,000 from his own company.

Domer, apparently calm, said that this must be a mistake in bookkeeping. If they would give him two days he was sure he could find the error. The investigators agreed. Domer then drove home, made a tape recording which he left for his wife, and disappeared.

While the police were turning up this information, Dr. Lester Adelson was completing his autopsy. He did not have very much to work with. There were only bits and pieces of burned flesh and bone, weighing a total of seventy-seven pounds. And these, Dr. Adelson noted, had already begun to smell. This seemed a bit unusual, but Dr. Adelson assumed that the heat of the fire and the fact that the remains had been wrapped in a plastic sheet had hastened the normal decomposition of the body.

Dr. Adelson found no CO (carbon monoxide) in the blood and no soot or carbon particles in the lungs. If the victim had been killed by the fire, even if he had drawn only three or four breaths, then in all probability there would have been CO in the blood and soot in the lungs. On the other hand, Dr. Adelson did find fat globules in the lungs, indicating that there was some circulation of blood at the time the body was touched by heat. At this point in his autopsy Adelson believed he was dealing with nothing more unusual than the victim of a crash and fire. He assumed, therefore, that the heat had been so sudden and so intense that it had caused a spasm of the larynx and this had prevented the victim from breathing. This, he figured, would account for the fact that there was no CO in the blood and no soot in the lungs.

The doctor's official decision was that the victim had died as the result of intense heat and flame.

There were two other items in the autopsy report that

the police found extremely interesting. The jaw had been badly burned, but there was enough left to show that all the teeth had been pulled sometime in the past. Also, the heart showed the scars of at least one serious heart attack.

The police now interviewed Robert Domer's personal doctor and his dentist. They learned that Domer, at the time of his disappearance, had never had a heart attack and never had his teeth pulled. So the body taken from the burning car could not have been that of Robert Domer.

The insurance companies were as interested in this fact as the police. Domer, it turned out, had insured his life for $288,000.

Five days after the crash, part of the mystery was solved. Robert Domer came home. His face and hands were badly burned and he wanted his wife to give him first aid. The police, who were watching his house, took him first to a doctor and then to jail.

He was willing to talk. He could hardly stop talking, even though his burned lips hurt when he spoke.

After the federal investigators had confronted him with the evidence of missing funds, Domer said, he had gone straight home and made the tape recording for his wife. Then he got in his automobile and began to drive. He didn't know where he was going and didn't care. He had no plan. He just drove, first in one direction, then another. He had drinks in various bars, spent the nights in motels. He used credit cards and cashed checks, some of them bad. In his three weeks of wandering he was never more than a few hundred miles from home. In fact, there were nights when he drove back and forth in front of his home, then went away again.

Fires and Strange Fuels

The police checked with Domer's bank, the credit card companies, bars, and motels. There could be no doubt that on this part of his story Robert Domer was telling the truth. Apparently he had been in a state of shock, making no real effort to hide the fact that he was still alive and close by.

Then he began to talk of what had happened in the last few days before the crash and fire.

He had been in a cheap bar in Akron, Ohio, Domer said. A tall, gaunt man, obviously drunk, had asked Domer to buy him a drink. Domer agreed. They talked. The man's name was Howard Riddle. He was obviously a bum, a wino, with no home, no relatives who might miss him. He and Domer moved from one bar to another. They spent the night in a motel, Domer paying the bill. For the next few days they rode about the country together with Riddle drunk most of the time.

Robert Domer may have been making plans. It is certain that several times he drove along the country road that crosses the Pennsylvania Railroad tracks west of Massillon. He learned something about train schedules.

Then it was April 21, two days before Pennsylvania train #50 would crash into Domer's flaming automobile. Domer and Howard Riddle were registered in a motel and Riddle was sick. Actually he had been sick for a couple of days, Domer said, vomiting much of the time but still drinking. On the night of the twenty-first, Domer went out to get some food, leaving Riddle asleep. When he came back he noticed that Riddle had not moved. His face had a strange look. Domer shook him—and stepped back in horror. Riddle was dead.

Science Catches the Criminal

At least this was Domer's story. He panicked, he said. Still in a state of shock, with no real plan for what he should do, Domer carried Riddle's body out of the motel and put it on the back seat of his car. He covered it with old newspapers and an overcoat. Then once more—it was not yet daylight of April 22—he began aimlessly driving.

But he was acutely conscious of the body on the back seat. What would happen if the police should recognize and stop him? Sometime during the day, Domer said, he checked into another motel. "I just sat there all day," he told the police. "I knew Mr. Riddle's body was in the car, and I went out repeatedly, but I couldn't look at it. I just went back and sat and sat and sat."

It was sometime during the afternoon, he said, that he decided to stage an accident and leave Riddle's body in the car, hoping it would be mistaken for his own.

About midnight he got in the automobile and drove to the nearest filling station. He bought a can of gasoline. Then he drove out to the lonely railroad crossing west of Massillon. He parked a few yards uphill from the tracks. It was now about two o'clock in the morning.

Domer knew that for Riddle's body to be mistaken for his own, it should be in the front seat. He uncovered it, and became more aware than ever that in the closed and heated car the body had begun to smell. But Domer pulled it out of the back seat and pushed it into the front. He put his wallet beside the body. He closed the door, leaving the window open, and stood there for a moment breathing hard.

Off to the east he heard the train and caught the first

glimpse of its headlight. Now he took the can of gasoline out of the trunk. He poured it over Riddle's body and the seat of the car. The train was coming faster than he had expected. He tossed the empty can into the ditch. He released the brakes on the automobile and it began to roll, slowly toward the tracks.

The train was almost on him now. He struck a match and flung it through the car window.

The automobile exploded like a bomb; and in almost the same instant it smashed into the train.

Robert Domer said he did not remember much after that. His face, neck, and hands were badly burned. The pain was so great he could not think. He did remember to carry the gasoline can some distance down the road. He kept walking until almost daylight, then hid. He was afraid to be seen with his burned face and hands. At night he started walking again. He stole scraps of food from garbage cans, and hid again. Five days after the wreck he came home, holding his burned hands out for his wife to bandage.

This was Domer's story. If it was true, then Domer was still guilty of embezzlement. But if it were not true, if Howard Riddle had been drunk but alive when Domer threw the match in the car, then Domer was guilty of murder.

Dr. Adelson's autopsy report said Riddle had been alive. The police charged Domer with murder and brought him to trial. Domer's attorney then called on Dr. Milton Helpern to testify for the defense.

Milton Helpern was the Chief Medical Examiner of the

Science Catches the Criminal

City of New York and one of the world's foremost authorities on forensic medicine. In his work he had personally performed more than 20,000 autopsies, many of them on the victims of violent crimes. He had either performed or personally supervised more than 2,000 autopsies on persons who had died by fire. Dr. Helpern had not performed the autopsy on Howard Riddle, but he had read Dr. Adelson's autopsy report. This autopsy, Helpern said, had been well and carefully done. He had no complaint on that score. Where the two doctors disagreed was on what these findings proved.

Dr. Adelson maintained that Riddle had been alive when the fire started. Dr. Helpern insisted that Adelson's own findings proved Riddle had been dead.

The jury was composed of laymen. They must accept the word of the one doctor or the other. Robert Domer's life depended on whom the jury believed.

Dr. Adelson testified first. He admitted that when a person was killed by fire there would, normally, be carbon monoxide in the blood and soot in the lungs. This was not true in Riddle's case. But Adelson explained this to the jury just as in his autopsy report: he believed that the sudden and intense heat of a gasoline fire had caused a spasm of the larynx. This prevented the victim from breathing, at least for a few moments, and within that time he died.

Then there was the decomposed condition of Riddle's body at the time of the autopsy. Dr. Adelson said frankly it was more putrefied than he would expect a body to become within twelve hours after death. But the fact that it had been destroyed by fire and wrapped in a plastic bag while still hot would account for this, he said.

104

Now it was Dr. Helpern's turn to testify. He explained that in the 2,000 autopsies he had performed on persons killed by fire there had not been a single one without carbon monoxide in the blood and soot in the lungs. This, he said, included many victims of airplane crashes where the fire had been as sudden and intense as that which destroyed Robert Domer's automobile.

Next was the condition of the body as Dr. Adelson had stated it in his autopsy. In discussing this, Dr. Helpern was asked to explain what happened when a living body died.

"The human body," Helpern said, "lives by way of its oxygen cycle. As long as this cycle is maintained the cells remain healthy . . . The body's chemical processes are maintained in balance so that its own self-destructive enzymes are neutralized . . . All self-destructive processes are held in check. Once, however, the oxygen cycle is interrupted by a cessation of breathing and circulation there is nothing left to hold these self-destructive enzymes in check."

When this happened, Helpern said, a "process known as putrefaction begins. This is an invasion of the various organs of the body structures by certain types of bacteria which are present in the intestinal tract . . . The bacteria thrive in a culture medium that no longer offers any resistance to their growth . . . The organs and soft tissues of the body liquify as the decaying process continues. So, instead of being reduced to dust, as the process has been graphically and poetically described, the body is turned into liquid and gas by its own enzymes and the invading bacteria."

How long, Helpern was asked, would it take a burned body to reach the condition described in Howard Riddle's autopsy. Could this take place within twelve hours?

Helpern shook his head. "Burned bodies simply do not decompose in this manner," he said. "This is the most important fact in the entire case . . . I would say from reading this autopsy that this suggests a process of about forty-eight hours, at least forty-eight hours . . . I can't fix the exact time . . . but I can say it was more than twenty-four hours and more in the area of forty-eight hours."

Here was a case in which two scientists differed by somewhere between twelve and thirty-six hours in estimating the time of death. Both men were honest, both extremely well trained. But under the law the jury, made up of persons with no scientific training at all, had to decide.

The jury decided that Howard Riddle had been alive when burned. Robert Domer was sentenced to death.

It was not the end of the case. Domer's attorney appealed to a higher court. The Court of Appeals was more impressed with Dr. Helpern's testimony than the jury had been. The Court ruled that "On the question of whether or not Riddle was alive when the fire started, as claimed by the State, with the many other facts developed in the record challenging such conclusion, it cannot be said that the State has shown the defendant caused the death of Riddle by incineration beyond a reasonable doubt."

Now the case had to be tried again. This time the jury, like the Court of Appeals, agreed with Helpern. Robert Domer went to prison for embezzlement, but not to the chair for murder.

Both Dr. Adelson and Dr. Helpern believed that, probably, they had been correct. Yet both recognized the other's view. After the case had been settled, Dr. Helpern often referred to it in classes of forensic medicine that he taught at both Cornell and New York University. "In many situations," he said, "the law demands more than medicine and medicine men can honestly give. Neither I nor anyone else can say with certainty what the real cause of death was. I believe it was a heart attack. There are some cases where a doctor can be absolutely sure. There are others where he can't."

In medical schools from coast to coast the case of Robert Domer is still discussed. And no one will ever know, with absolute certainty, what is right.

Suicide? Suicide!

A policeman in the Tottenham Court Road Police Station in London, England, sat staring at the letter in his hands. He shook his head, then read the letter a second and third time. Finally he took it to his superior officer and put it on the desk. "This just came in the mail," he said.

The inspector read it.

Dear Sir,

You will be mystified by an accident occuring in Hampstead Road area, involving fire which you may suspect to be murder, but is simply Sucide. I'm sorry for any damage or trouble I may cause. Fortunately I have no relatives in south England to fret.

Now it was the inspector's turn to shake his head. "What do you make of it?" he asked.

"Well, sir, I've read some suicide notes. But this doesn't sound like one."

"The word *suicide* is misspelled. That might be the result of tension, or ignorance, or . . ."

"The note might be a wonderful cover for somebody planning a murder."

"Just what I was thinking," the inspector said. "Do we have any dead bodies lying around that this might apply to?"

"Not at present."

"Well, keep an eye out."

The police did not have long to wait. This was in 1951 and there were still a number of buildings that had been bombed out during the war and not yet rebuilt. On the day after the "suicide note," one of these caught fire. When the blaze was brought under control firemen found the remains of what had been a man. The body lay on its back, the charred arms raised as if clawing the air—a condition quite common where death is the result of fire. Near the head, from which the face had burned completely away, were two empty cans.

If some murderer had hoped that an apparent suicide note would keep the police from making a thorough investigation, then he was wrong. Instead, because of the note, the Scotland Yard pathologists worked even harder than usual.

Tests showed that the two cans found near the body had held paraffin. The body itself had been soaked with paraffin from head to foot. And death had surely been the result of fire: the lungs were black with soot, the blood heavy with carbon monoxide. Nor could the doctors find any other possible cause of death. Until the moment the fire began, the man had apparently been in excellent health.

The body, the burned clothing, the charred floor beneath the body were all inspected minutely. A needle and a razor blade were found in the burned clothing. But there were no narcotics in the body, no alcohol, no sign that the man had been made unconscious before the fire. Nor were there any charred bits of rope or wire to indicate he might have been tied.

Days passed and no one came forward to report a missing person who might possibly have been the dead man.

The Department of Anatomy at Guy's Hospital now took thirty X-ray photographs of the skull, viewing it from every angle. Precise measurements were made, not only of the skull but of the amounts of tissue that covered parts of it. From these a wax head was built with a face that must have closely resembled that of the dead man. A photograph of this was circulated throughout England.

But if the photo really resembled the dead man, the police never knew for sure. He was never identified, and until this day the case remains a mystery.

The Overdone Undertaker

Let's call the two men Smith and Jones. These are not their true names, but the rest of the story is true.

Smith and Jones had an undertaking establishment in Upstate New York. Business was good and profits were good. But there was a racetrack nearby and both Smith and Jones were hooked on horses. They gambled steadily; sometimes they won, but more often they lost. They borrowed money against their business—and saw it dribble away.

Smith took out a $100,000 life insurance policy on Jones, payable to Smith. Jones took out a similar policy on Smith. Both were double indemnity; this is, in case either Smith or Jones was accidentally killed, the policy would pay double. Such policies are rather common among business partners and at the time no one thought much of it.

About this same time, the partners bought a small fishing cabin on a trout stream in the Adirondack Mountains. Neither Smith nor Jones had ever shown much interest in fishing; but habits change, and again no one paid much attention.

The spring and summer passed. Occasionally Smith or Jones would spend a weekend at their fishing cabin, though they rarely went together. Then one beautiful autumn morning a young couple, wandering through the woods to look at the colored leaves, saw a column of smoke and fire above the trees. They hurried forward and found a cabin—they did not even know who owned it—a mass of roaring flames.

There was an automobile in the cabin yard, but no keys in it. The young couple raced to the nearby highway, flagged down the first passing auto, and asked the driver to report the fire.

It was only a few minutes before a fire truck arrived from the resort town a few miles down the road. It was much too late to save the cabin, but the firemen put out the blaze to keep it from spreading to the trees. Peering into the still-hot embers, the firemen saw what seemed to be the remains of a human body. As soon as possible these remains were gathered up and carried to the nearest undertaking establishment.

A telephone check with the courthouse supplied the names of the cabin's owners. A call was made, and it was Smith who rushed to the scene. He looked at the burned remains, shivered slightly, and said it was totally impossible to identify what was here. He did, however, identify the automobile in the cabin yard as that belonging to his partner Jones. The car keys, which had been found with the burned body, also belonged to Jones. And Jones, Mr. Smith said, had told him he planned to spend the weekend at the cabin. Sorrowfully, he announced there could be little doubt that his friend Jones had been destroyed by fire. This meant that the insurance company owed Smith $200,-000.

Meanwhile, the local fire chief and his assistant had been poking about among the still-warm cabin ashes. Theirs was a small fire department, but it served a rather wealthy community and was well equipped. Both men knew their business.

"Just where," the chief asked his assistant, "do you think the fire started?"

When wood burns it tends to char in a pattern of rough rectangles, somewhat like the bony plates on an alligator's back. And near the fire's origin these get smaller and smaller until they crumble into ash all together.

Science Catches the Criminal

The assistant chief pointed toward what had been the cabin's window. "It looks as if it started somewhere in this area."

"That's what I was thinking," the chief said. "Only it doesn't make sense. The fireplace is on the other side of the room. There's no stove, no electric wiring over here. So what started the fire?"

The assistant said he would go and fetch the Snifter.

The Snifter's more formal name is the J-W Automatic Hydrocarbon Indicator. It was invented originally to detect dangerous gases in factories and mines, and is so sensitive that it can pick up and record one part in a hundred thousand. It is light enough to be easily moved from place to place, and fire departments were quick to make use of it in cases of suspected arson.

Held where the window of the cabin had been, the Snifter's needle wavered slightly. Lowered to the ground, the needle really jumped. "If somebody stood outside the cabin and poured kerosene or gasoline inside the window," the fire chief said, "they might well have spilled some outside."

"Yes, sir," the assistant said. He carefully dug up some of the dirt and put it in a box to send to the laboratory.

Smith, the undertaker, knew nothing of what the firemen were doing. He applied to the insurance company for his $200,000. The insurance company stalled; they asked for an autopsy on the remains found in the cabin.

About this time the laboratory reported on the dirt above which the Snifter's needle had wavered. The dirt contained kerosene. It was not enough so that a human nose would ever have noticed it, but the Snifter had caught the scent.

The fire chief reported that in his opinion the cabin had been deliberately set afire.

Next day came the autopsy report. The torso of the corpse had been fairly intact after the fire. The lungs showed no trace of soot, so the victim had not been alive when the fire started. What the lungs did show was that the man had suffered from acute pneumonia; in fact, he probably had died as the result of pneumonia. This seemed odd, since Jones had apparently set out to go fishing while in excellent health. Moreover, various body organs contained large amounts of formaldehyde, a principal constituent of embalming fluid.

There was still another item. The long bones of the dead man's right leg were charred, but intact. Working with these, the pathologists estimated his height at not less than five-feet-eleven inches. The missing Jones had been five-feet-eight.

The police now began to search the records of the Smith and Jones undertaking establishment. They found where, quite recently, they had buried a man named Thomas. Mr. Thomas had been five-feet-eleven and one-half inches tall, and had died of acute pneumonia. His family had requested a closed casket, and so no one had seen the body after it was taken by the undertakers.

The Thomas casket was dug up. It contained wet sand and rocks, nothing else.

Confronted with all this, Smith admitted that he and Jones had planned to defraud the insurance company. Jones was found hiding in another cabin some two hundred miles away. And both men went to prison.

7

WATER IN THE HEART

The Brides in the Bath

His real name was Smith—George Joseph Smith—though he rarely used it. He came to his end suddenly, at the end of a rope, more than half a century ago; yet his story remains one of the classics of forensic medicine and is used today in medical schools.

Even before his trial for murder, Smith had been made famous—or infamous—by British newspapers in what was called The Brides in the Bath story. Almost everyone in England felt certain that Smith was guilty, not only of one murder, but of three and possibly more. At the same time, almost everyone believed he would be found not guilty. British law requires that a jury be convinced beyond "a reasonable doubt." And George Joseph Smith had invented a new kind of murder.

The man called on to prove *how* Smith committed his murders was a young doctor named Bernard Spilsbury. Later he would be known as The Scalpel of Scotland Yard, the most famous practitioner of forensic medicine in all England, and the terror of criminals. But in 1915, when

114

Smith came to trial, Spilsbury was little known outside his own profession.

Bernard Spilsbury was tall, rather handsome in a heavy, extremely dignified sort of way. He spoke in tones of such authority that he often annoyed even the people who understood and admired his ability. There were those who said Spilsbury advanced his opinions like Moses handing down the Ten Commandments. None of this bothered the doctor: he lived in and for his work.

George Joseph Smith was something else. Born into an average, honest, middle-class family, he got into such repeated trouble that he was sent to a reformatory when nine years old. By the time he was eighteen he was out of the reformatory, but back in jail for stealing.

In his early twenties Smith married for the first time. He forged such excellent letters of reference for his wife, even though she had almost no education, that she was able to get a good job. Then Smith taught her how to steal from her employers. She was caught—but she was one of the few women in Smith's career who got some revenge. She told the police that her husband had been taking and selling what she stole, and once more Smith went to jail.

Released, George Joseph Smith decided that it was too dangerous to have women steal for him. Instead, he would steal from them. From this time on, women were Smith's career.

To Bernard Spilsbury, and to all the men who later learned what Smith was doing, the whole thing seemed incredible, impossible. Men regarded Smith as repulsive looking. He had a long, bony face, a narrow jaw, thin lips, a moth-eaten mustache. But the dominant feature was his eyes. They were black and they glittered. Later, the lawyer who defended Smith referred to his "horrible way of looking at me." This lawyer believed that Smith's glittering eyes hypnotized the women he encountered. Spilsbury did not agree. But whatever the reason, Smith repulsed men and fascinated women. Even when he was being tried for murder, women crowded into the courtroom to stare at him, to try to touch him. They went home and wrote him letters.

Smith quite obviously recognized his talents and he picked the women on whom they were most effective. He wandered about England, particularly around seaside resorts, picking up women. Sometimes he married them, using a variety of names; sometimes a day or two of courting was enough for him to move in. But he rarely stayed more than a few weeks—just long enough to learn what jewels and clothing his victim owned, and to get her to withdraw any money she had in the bank.

Next, Smith used a technique that is difficult to understand. He must have done it through deliberate cruelty, some deep hatred for the women he victimized. It would have been easy enough to wait until the woman was away from home, then steal her possessions and disappear. Instead, he usually took her on some sort of lovers' treat: a walk in the park where they had met, a dinner in a particular restaurant. Then he excused himself for a moment, went back to the house or apartment, and cleaned it out. He took everything, of value or not, leaving his lady love with nothing except the clothing she wore while patiently waiting for him to return.

How many women Smith married, or pretended to marry, was never determined. The odds are that Smith himself could not remember them all. Among them was just one for whom he seemed to feel any affection. Her name was Edith Pegler. For the last seven years of his life Smith lived with her, off and on. He was always going on mysterious journeys; once he left her for a full year and in that time sent her five dollars to live on. But he always came back.

When the story of Smith and The Brides in the Bath was appearing in every British newspaper, a reporter asked Edith Pegler if Smith himself bathed often. She had to think before she answered. In the past seven years, she said, Smith had taken only one bath she knew of. Indeed, on one occasion when she was about to step into the bathtub, Smith had cautioned her against it. Women, he said, had been known to die in bathtubs, of heart failure and other troubles.

This was a subject on which Smith had, quietly and with practice, made himself an authority. For some fifteen years he had lived off women while committing no crime more violent than theft. Even so, most of the women he met had little to steal. Perhaps he was growing impatient.

In the summer of 1910, using the name Williams, he met a thirty-three-year-old woman named Bessie Mundy. She was neither pretty nor smart, but she told "Williams" that she owned some $12,000 in gilt-edged stock. Almost instantly he proposed. A few days later they were married.

Then, in frustrated anger, Smith learned that Bessie's father had long since realized that she was incapable of looking after her own money. The $12,000 was tied up in a trust and she could draw only the interest.

There was, however, some $600 she could withdraw from the bank. She did so, at Smith's urging. Then he took her to visit the art gallery where they had met. There he left her to look at the pictures while he went to the washroom.

She did not see or hear from him again for almost two years, except for one very nasty letter. Whether he met her again by accident or design is uncertain. Probably it was just bad luck for Bessie. She had gone to a seaside resort named Weston. Walking along the beach one day she came face to face with her long lost husband. He looked at her with his glittering black eyes, said he had missed her terribly, and they went back to her hotel together.

This was in March of 1912. A few weeks later Mr. and Mrs. Williams were in a place called Herne Bay. There Smith called on a lawyer with a theoretical question: suppose a woman owned a trust fund which she could not withdraw. But suppose this woman died, leaving all her property to her husband. Would he then be able to get the money? The lawyer said yes.

Thoughtfully, Smith walked back to the house where the loving but stupid Bessie was waiting.

On July 8, Smith and Bessie Mundy executed wills, leaving everything they owned to one another. On July 9, Smith sent his wife out to buy a bathtub. He told her to buy the cheapest one possible, but it must be long enough to lie down in. And she should buy it on credit. Bessie did as she was told.

On July 10, Smith and Bessie went to a doctor. His wife, Smith said, had fainting spells. She didn't remember fainting, but accepted her husband's word for it. The doctor gave her some medicine and sent her home.

On July 12, the same doctor was called to the Williams' house. Bessie had a violent headache. (Later Dr. Spilsbury and the police would wonder about the headaches that all of Smith's brides had before their final baths. Were they the result of hypnotism? A lick on the head? Some drug given to them? Spilsbury was inclined to believe it was a drug; but by the time he met the brides it was too late for him to determine.) The doctor gave Bessie some more medicine and then went home.

Early the very next morning the doctor received a note. It read: "Can you come at once? I am afraid my wife is dead."

She was certainly dead by the time the doctor got there. She was still in the bathtub, her face underwater. A bar of soap was clutched tightly in her right hand.

Williams told the doctor that he'd been outside the house that morning. When he came in he found his wife here, in the tub. He had been afraid to move her. He knew that in the past she'd had epileptic fits, fainting fits.

It was a Saturday morning. (All of Smith's brides would die on either a Friday night or Saturday morning.) The doctor was in a hurry. He said the death was due to drowning during an epileptic fit.

George Joseph Smith was never a man to waste money

119

on other persons. He had Bessie buried in a pauper's grave at government expense. He sent the tub back to the store from which it had been bought on credit. He collected his $12,000 trust fund, and vanished.

In October, 1913, a rather pretty girl named Alice Burnham, a professional nurse, was taking a vacation at Southsea. On Sunday she went to church and sitting next to her was a man with glittering black eyes whom she found intensely attractive. They exchanged glances, whispered words, read from the same prayer book. When the service was over they walked out together.

Alice Burnham was a far more intelligent girl than Bessie Mundy had been. Even so, she found her new friend—he was using his real name of Smith—irresistible. She told him she had a little money of her own and some jewelry, and he found her irresistible also.

Alice took her friend home to meet her father, who found Smith repulsive. He warned his daughter to have nothing to do with Smith. Yet within a month after they met, Alice and Smith were married.

Smith learned that Alice had loaned her father money. He wrote threatening letters to Mr. Burnham demanding that the loan be repaid. At the same time he took his new bride out and had her insured for $2,500, after which they went to Blackpool for a honeymoon.

It was very brief. Alice immediately had a headache. She and her husband went to a doctor who found nothing seriously wrong. But next day Alice was dead in her bathtub. It was Friday night and no real time for an inquest. The doctor decided that Alice had fainted as a result of the headaches and hot water, then drowned. By the time Alice's father had been notified and could reach the scene, Alice had been buried in a pauper's grave. "When they're dead, they're dead," Smith remarked. He collected his insurance and vanished, leaving Mr. Burnham mystified, furious, but helpless.

During the next year Smith robbed various women of small sums, but none of them seem to have been worth killing. Then, in December, 1914, almost exactly one year after Alice Burnham's death, he met a lonely, thirty-eight-year-old woman named Margaret Lofty. Margaret told him her life was insured for $3,500. Smith proposed, and he took his lady friend to—of all places—a town named Bath to be married.

Smith was now using the name of Lloyd. "Mr. Lloyd" and Miss Lofty were married on December 17. That same afternoon Mrs. Lloyd came down with such a headache it was necessary to see a doctor. She felt better the next morning, well enough to go with her new husband to visit a lawyer and make wills. And at 7:30 that same evening the bride took a bath.

They were staying in a rooming house. The landlady heard a splashing in the bathtub on the second floor, but thought little of it. A few minutes later she heard Mr. Lloyd playing the organ in the living room. He played "Nearer My God to Thee." After he quit there was a brief pause. Then Mr. Lloyd appeared at his landlady's door to ask, quite calmly, if she would come with him: he had just found his wife in the bathtub with her face underwater and he was afraid she was dead.

Science Catches the Criminal

She was.

Again things went smoothly for Smith, at least through the doctor's report and the burial. But then, finally, his luck began to run out.

The newspapers reported on the tragic death of the bride in her bath at Bath. It wasn't a large story, but back in the town of Aston Clinton it caught the eye of Mr. Charles Burnham, Alice's father. Mr. Burnham had been suspicious of George Joseph Smith from the time he laid eyes on him. He had been even more suspicious after Alice's death. And now there was this story of another bride drowning in her tub, matching the story of his daugther's death in every detail.

Mr. Burnham wrote the police. The police began to investigate. It didn't take twenty-four hours to realize that they were on to something.

There was one problem. Smith, as usual, had disappeared. The insurance company, however, had not yet paid off. So the police merely waited, and when "Mr. John Lloyd" showed up to collect, they grabbed him.

In prison, Smith admitted having robbed a few women. There were too many witnesses to do otherwise. But he was, Smith insisted, innocent of murder. And he had the statement of the three different doctors who had attended his brides to back him up. Each death was listed as accidental. Also, two of the deaths had taken place in rooming houses occupied by other persons. It seemed impossible that a man could drown a full-grown woman in a tub without a struggle or sounds that would alert persons nearby.

This was the situation when Dr. Bernard Spilsbury was called into the case.

By now police had located all three of the drowned brides. Their bodies were exhumed and taken to the laboratory at St. Mary's Hospital in London where Spilsbury did most of his work.

It was long, slow, tedious work. By now two of the bodies, poorly embalmed, were badly decomposed.

Spilsbury's first job was to determine whether or not the women had actually drowned. In doing this he used criteria partly worked out by Dr. Sydney Smith who had studied many cases of drowning in Egypt.

Was there a fine, frothy foam in the mouth and nose? Was similar foam in the windpipe and bronchial tubes? Were the lungs overinflated and soggy? Was there water in the stomach?

None of these were absolute proof of drowning, but together they added up to the best proof known in 1915. And there was one other point. Dr. Smith had observed that many drowning persons clutched violently at any available object and held to it, even after death.

Bessie Mundy had died holding a bar of soap so tightly it had been difficult to take it from her hand. There was froth in her nose, windpipe, and bronchial tubes, and this was also true of the other brides. Spilsbury concluded they had all drowned.

But how? Spilsbury's first theory was the women had been made unconscious by some type of drug, then held underwater. But test after test for drugs failed. If they had been drugged, Spilsbury could find no evidence of it. Nor could he find any injury that suggested they had been knocked unconscious. On one body he found several small bruises underneath the skin. These must have been caused immediately before death, Spilsbury reasoned; otherwise there would have been time for them to show on the skin.

Spilsbury sent for the bathtub in which Alice Burnham had drowned. The tub was five feet long. Alice Burnham had been five-feet-five inches tall. It would be natural for such a person to bathe with head and shoulders resting on the sloping end of the tub above the water.

The landlady who had helped Smith take Alice Burnham's body out of the tub said that Alice's feet and lower legs had stretched across the foot of the tub, outside. This was the same condition in which Bessie Mundy and Margaret Lofty had been found. It seemed like a very unnatural way to bathe, particularly for a woman who might not want to get her hair wet.

Spilsbury knew that a person snatched underwater without warning, so that water is forced into the nose and mouth, may lose consciousness almost instantly. He asked one of the hospital nurses, who was also an excellent swimmer, to help him with an experiment.

With other doctors and police watching, they filled Alice Burnham's tub with water. Wearing a bathing suit, the nurse stepped in. She sat leaning her head and shoulders against the back of the tub as she might have if bathing.

Spilsbury knelt beside the tub. He slid his left arm under the nurse's bent knees. He put his right hand on her head. A man pretending to be about to lift his wife from the tub might have been in just such a position.

Suddenly Spilsbury raised his left arm, jerking the nurse's knees and feet clear of the water. At the same time he pushed down with his right hand, shoving her head below the surface.

The nurse had known what Spilsbury planned to do, but not the exact moment. She gasped, flung her arms wildly about, and went unconscious. She was lifted quickly from the tub and it took artificial respiration to bring her around.

After this the police were sure of their ground. They brought George Joseph Smith to trial, and Spilsbury to the witness stand. Point by point he destroyed every argument the defense could advance.

Smith claimed that Bessie Mundy had epileptic fits. Her family said she had never been known to have fits. Spilsbury testified that it would be very exceptional for a woman of Bessie's age to develop epilepsy. But if she had, Spilsbury said, her body would have stiffened; her feet, against the foot of the tub, would push her head and shoulders *up*, well clear of the water. Nor had she simply fainted. In that case all her muscles would have gone slack; she would not have been found clutching a bar of soap so tightly it was difficult to straighten her fingers.

Spilsbury testified that his autopsies had shown that all Smith's brides had been healthy. None had died of a heart attack; they had drowned. Also, he could show how—and he did. He gave his evidence in such deliberate, ponderous tones that all the jury, and everyone else listening, was totally convinced.

Questioned by both the prosecution and defense, it took Spilsbury two days to complete his testimony. It took the jury twenty minutes to find George Joseph Smith guilty and sentence him to hang.

Fresh Water, or Salt?

Almost every specialist in forensic medicine has, at one time or another, been presented with a body found in water and the question: was this person drowned, or was he already dead, then thrown in the water?

For years the best criteria to determine drowning was that developed by Dr. Sydney Smith and used by Spilsbury in sending George Joseph Smith to the gallows: a fine, frothy foam in the mouth and nose; foam in the bronchial tubes and windpipe; foreign material clutched in the hands; soggy lungs; water in the stomach.

No one of these things was absolute evidence in itself. On the other hand, there were many cases of drowning where not all of them were present. Some better method of knowing, surely, whether or not a person had drowned was needed.

In 1921 Dr. Alexander Gettler, Chief Toxicologist for the New York City Medical Examiner's office, came up with the answer.

Dr. Gettler knew that a drowning person makes a long, desperate effort to hold his breath. It is believed that this is an automatic reaction even with a person trying to commit suicide. But there comes a time within seconds, or within two or three minutes at the most, when the person must try to breathe. Then water is sucked into the lungs.

And the lungs, Dr. Gettler knew, are closely connected to the *left side* of the heart through the great pulmonary vein. So water from the lungs will slowly seep into the left side of the heart, diluting the blood.

On the other hand, if a dead body is thrown into the water there is no desperate gulping for air; no water is sucked deep into the lungs; and no water at all will find its way into the heart. Therefore, water in the heart meant drowning. No water in the heart meant the body was dead before it went into the water.

Carefully, Dr. Gettler checked his theory. He used animals known to have drowned, and animals destroyed in the laboratory, then put in water. He used human bodies where the circumstances of the death were known. And in every case, without exception, his theory proved correct.

Now Dr. Gettler took his test one step farther. Human blood contains some salt. If a body drowned in fresh water that contained little or no salt, then the diluted blood of the heart would contain less than the normal amount of salt. But ocean water is saltier than blood. So if the blood in the left side of the heart was saltier than normal, the drowning had been in salt water.

Again Dr. Gettler checked and rechecked his tests on known cases. Soon they were accepted by scientific detectives all over the world.

Then one case blew up.

The body of a small boy was brought to Dr. Gettler's laboratory. The boy had been seen to fall through the ice while skating on a freshwater pond. But in New York all accidental deaths require an autopsy.

Dr. Gettler performed the autopsy and wrote his report: death by drowning in salt water.

A doctor who knew about the case from the first called Gettler. "There is a mistake on your report. You said salt water."

"That's right."

"But it was a freshwater pond," the doctor said. "I helped recover the body. I live close by. I know this is a freshwater pond."

"I'll check my findings," Gettler said.

He checked, time after time. And every test showed salt water.

Some person might have shrugged and forgotten the matter. Not Dr. Gettler. He lived by science, and now science seemed to be playing tricks.

Gettler went to the pond where the boy had drowned, cut a hole through the ice near the middle, and tested the water. It was fresh. But still Gettler did not quit. He started to ask questions of everybody who lived nearby.

"Well," a grocery store owner told him, "the only thing I can think of is this. I did have a barrel of salt that got dirt spilled in it. I couldn't sell the salt. So I poured it into the pond. As I remember, that was just the day before the weather turned cold and the pond froze."

Gettler asked where in the pond he had poured the salt. It was exactly the same spot where the boy had drowned. And finally Dr. Gettler understood how the child had drowned in salt water in a freshwater pond. His tests were still accurate.

8

DEADLY POISON

On Their Wedding Eve

A young couple died on their wedding eve. Later, two other persons came within a hair's-breadth of dying. A girl's career was ruined because of wild gossip. Two families that had been friends turned into bitter enemies, and a whole town was divided against itself.

The chain of events began on the last day of 1910 in Cumberland, Maryland. It could have been only yesterday in almost any small town—if the doctor was a little careless with no training in forensic medicine.

On December 31, 1910, a young man named Charles Edward Twigg went to call on his fiancée, Grace Elosser. Grace lived with her mother and younger sister, and though both these women liked Charles, they were not too happy to see him at the moment. He and Grace were to be married the next day and the Elosser household was in the usual state of confusion that precedes a wedding.

Charles and Grace went into the living room and Grace closed the door. This was partially for privacy, partially because the day was cold and the old house was heated by stoves or fireplaces in the various rooms. Mrs. Elosser and May, her younger daughter, went about their work.

An hour or so passed. Mrs. Elosser needed to ask Grace a question about the wedding and opened the living room door. The young couple was sitting close together on the sofa. Charles had his arm around Grace, her head resting on his shoulder. Mrs. Elosser closed the door softly, knocked, waited a few seconds, and opened the door again. The couple had not moved.

"Grace," Mrs. Elosser said. Then, "Grace!" She went closer, touched her daughter on the shoulder, and began to scream.

May came running. She and her mother half-carried, half-dragged Grace into an adjoining bedroom and put her on the bed. They rubbed her wrists, put smelling salts under her nose. Then the sister went racing out of the house and down the street to the office of Dr. W. H. Foard, a few blocks away.

The doctor wasted no time, but there was nothing he could do. He was still bending over Grace's body, listening for a heartbeat, when Dr. G. L. Broadrupp arrived. The two doctors looked at one another and shook their heads. They gave Mrs. Elosser, who was on the verge of hysterics, a sedative.

Dr. Foard had been in the house about ten minutes, Dr. Broadrupp perhaps five minutes, when May Elosser said to them, "Look at what we have in here," and pointed to the living room. Charles Twigg was still sitting on the sofa, his arm curved just as it had been around Grace's shoulders. And he, like Grace, was dead.

The bodies were sent to the local coroner for autopsies. The coroner found nothing unusual; there was a bit of chewing gum in Charles' mouth, but it was known that he often chewed gum. Neither Dr. Foard nor Broadrupp could explain the cause of death, so the contents of the stomachs were turned over to a local chemist.

On January 2, the chemist announced his findings. Both stomachs had traces of potassium cyanide.

The news hit the small town of Cumberland like a bomb. Everybody had heard of potassium cyanide. It had the most fearsome reputation of any known poison. The smallest touch to the lips was supposed to bring almost instant death. But how had it been given, and by whom? Was this a double murder? A murder and suicide? A double suicide? Rumors galloped like wild horses up and down the streets of Cumberland.

One of the first and most widely held theories was that the cyanide had been on the gum in Charles' mouth. Then he had kissed Grace, and the touch of his poisoned lips had instantly killed her. This theory was strengthened by the fact there had been a larger trace of cyanide in Charles' stomach than in Grace's. Also, the police found a pack of gum with one stick missing in Grace Elosser's room.

But who put the cyanide on the gum?

On the street corners, in the local drug and grocery stores, people remembered that Charles had known Grace for only about four months. In fact, he had met her sister May before he met Grace. May and Charles had gone riding together in his buggy. Soon it was whispered, then said aloud, that May had been in love with Charles, who had deserted her for Grace. And it would have been easy for May to put the cyanide on the gum in Grace's room. She had planned to kill Grace, the gossips said, but Grace had given the gum to Charles who put it in his mouth, kissed Grace, and both died.

Within twenty-four hours gossip had convicted May Elosser of double murder.

Both Dr. Foard and Dr. Broadrupp knew more about potassium cyanide than did the general public of Cumberland. They knew that pure prussic or hydrocyanic acid can cause almost instant death. They knew also that this pure product is unavailable except in a very few laboratories. The more common potassium cyanide, closely related to the pure prussic acid, is also deadly, but not in such minute quantities. In fact, it was commonly used in some silver polish, in photography, and in various industries. It was, therefore, available to the person who really sought it. But to kill, it would require more than an invisible grain or two upon a stick of gum.

The doctors accepted the chemist's report that potassium cyanide had caused the deaths. However, they thought it had probably been given in some liquid.

This, Mrs. Elosser said, was impossible. There had been no glass, no bottle, nothing in the room that could have held such a liquid. May backed her mother's statement.

Gossip, that had already convicted May of the murder, whispered that Mrs. Elosser was protecting her daughter. Charles Twigg's family felt certain that Charles had been killed by some Elosser, though they didn't know which. And the Elossers felt equally certain that, somehow, Charles had killed Grace. On January 3, when both Charles and Grace were buried, no Twigg was at Grace's funeral. No Elosser was present to mourn Charles.

On the next day the story took a new, sinister turn. An eight-year-old boy named Harlan Norris went to the police. He lived only a few doors from the Elossers and had been walking past their house, he said, when he saw the daughter May running down the street. She was waving her arms and calling for a doctor. Curious, the boy had walked up on the Elosser front porch and looked through the window. He saw Charles and Grace sitting stiffly on the sofa. Charles had a jelly glass in his hand; Grace held a small wine glass. On the floor at Charles' feet was a pint milk bottle half-filled with a greenish liquid. Mrs. Elosser was standing beside Grace, shaking her and crying.

The sight, Harlan Norris said, held him frozen against the window. He was there when Dr. Foard entered, running past the boy without seeing him. He took the glasses from the hands of the dead couple, said something to Mrs. Elosser, who cried, "This must be hushed up!"

This all frightened young Harlan so badly, he said, that he had run home, and for several days had not mentioned what he saw. Then he told his mother, and she sent him to the police.

Mrs. Elosser said the whole story was a lie. Dr. Foard said that the hands of both Grace and Charles had been empty but clinched tight when he found them. This clinching of the fingers would be natural after sudden death. But if anyone had opened their hands to remove glasses, Dr. Foard said, the fingers would have remained open and flexible until rigor mortis set in. Yet their hands had still been clinched when Dr. Broadrupp arrived. Dr. Broadrupp agreed with Dr. Foard.

A coroner's jury brought a verdict of murder by persons unknown.

And here, for awhile, the case ended—except for gossip and newspaper stories. The gossip centered on May Elosser, a small, quiet girl, a schoolteacher who could no longer face the staring eyes of her pupils. She stayed in her room, the blinds pulled. And slowly, in the back of her mind, she began to wonder if, somehow, she had caused her sister's death.

The newspapers continued to publish stories. Reporters had come from all over the country. Rewards were offered for a solution to the mystery.

Two doctors named J. R. Littlefield and A. H. Hawkins read the stories and became fascinated with the case. It was not the reward that interested them, but the mystery. They read the autopsy report and they went to see the chemist who had analyzed the contents of the dead couple's stomachs.

They learned that although he had found traces of potassium cyanide, he had made no test to determine the amount. Doctors Littlefield and Hawkins pointed out that potassium cyanide is always present in the human stomach, in very minute amounts. A test that did not determine the amount was of no value.

Littlefield and Hawkins studied the autopsy reports again, then turned to the weather reports. December 31 had been a cold day. The doctors went to the Elosser home, looked over the living room where the couple had died, and went away.

When they came back they had two cats in a cage. They put the cage on the sofa where Charles Twigg and Grace Elosser had once sat. They lit a fire in the natural gas stove that heated the room, closed the windows and left, carefully closing the door behind them.

They waited two hours. They opened the windows of the living room from outside, then opened the door and went in. The cats looked as if they were peacefully sleeping, but they were dead.

"So that's it," Dr. Littlefield said to Dr. Hawkins. "That gas stove isn't properly vented. They died of carbon monoxide poisoning."

The experiment was repeated for the police, with the doctors explaining. Natural gas contains carbon monoxide. When this gas is burned in a stove with defective vents, the carbon monoxide may escape in the room. If windows or doors are open, the gas may blow away, causing no damage. But if there is no ventilation, the gas collects. A person breathing it for a relatively short time may have a headache, or feel dizzy, and nothing more. A long exposure to small amounts of carbon monoxide may make a person act as if drunk, stumbling around and falling over things. But a heavy concentration of carbon monoxide kills very quietly, the victim merely drifting off to sleep, and never awakening.

When Mrs. Elosser entered her living room to speak to Grace, she left the door open. She was there only a few moments before carrying Grace's body to a bedroom. By the time the doctors were shown into the living room the gas had blown away.

Police accepted the explanation of Doctors Littlefield and Hawkins, but the gossips still whispered that May Elosser had murdered her sister. May and Mrs. Elosser stood it for a while. The stove's vent had been cleaned of soot, making it temporarily safe. But after a year Mrs. Elosser sold the house and moved away.

The new owners were two old ladies. On a cold day a neighbor came to call. She knocked, got no answer, and looked in the window. The old ladies were sitting in the living room, motionless, staring into space.

The neighbor jerked open the door, rushed in, threw open windows, and called for help. The old ladies were revived. Now, finally, the stove was dismantled, the flue carefully examined. And it was discovered that improperly placed bricks in the flue collected soot which in time blocked the flue, letting the carbon monoxide escape back into the room.

Even the worst of the gossips had trouble blaming this on May Elosser who was now several hundred miles away.

Cherry Red

There is a strange similarity between deaths caused by carbon monoxide and those caused by cyanide poisoning. In both cases the skin of the victim will often turn cherry red, or at least be splotched by red markings. This may have added to the problems of Doctors Foard and Broadrupp in dealing with the Elosser deaths, though they made no mention of it. But with medical examiners trained in forensic medicine this coloration of the skin has sometimes pointed directly to either murder or innocence.

It was on the day before Christmas that Dr. Edward Marten, Deputy Chief Medical Examiner of New York City, was called by the police. The address given was an apartment building in a poor section. The apartment itself was barely furnished, but clean. In one bedroom a woman lay dead. Her husband and two policemen were standing by. From another bedroom came the sound of children crying.

The husband was a tall, thin man. He wore a suit that had once been fashionable but now was old and threadbare. His face was tear-stained. "It must have been a heart attack," he told Dr. Marten. And repeated, "Her heart. It must have been her heart."

Looking down at the woman's body, Dr. Marten had other ideas. Her face and throat were unnaturally red. Marten looked around to see how the room was heated; it was a hot water radiator, not gas. "Is this where you found her?" he asked.

"Yes," the husband said. "Only a half hour ago. I called an ambulance . . ."

Marten leaned close and with his right hand lifted the woman's eyelid. As he did, his left forearm rested on her chest. This forced a little air from her lungs and Dr. Marten caught a sharp odor like that of peach seeds. He recognized it instantly: potassium cyanide. Turning to the husband, he snapped, "What are you trying to pull on us? This was no heart attack!"

The man began to sob. But it was not murder, he confessed. This was during the Great Depression of the 1930's. The husband had been a well-to-do jewler, but had lost his job. He had moved his family from their former home into a cheap apartment. Still, his savings disappeared little by little. Now they were all gone. There was no money for Christmas presents for the children. Two days before Christmas his wife had stolen dolls from a department store, meaning to give them to her little girls. She had been caught. The judge had let her go home for Christmas, but she was to be tried later. It was something she could not face. There was potassium cyanide in the house; her husband had used it often in his jewelry business. And she had killed herself.

Such a story might not have been believable at other times. But during the Depression when men were out of work everywhere and whole families going hungry, Dr. Marten did believe. A police check proved it to be true. And Dr. Marten went slowly home, wondering if perhaps it had been better if he had not recognized the cherry red skin of cyanide or carbon monoxide poisoning and had let the death pass as a simple heart attack.

In his work as medical examiner Dr. Edward Marten would soon have another case in which he had no doubts about right and wrong. In this case he was called to a dirty tenement apartment on the east side of New York. Here, as before, a woman lay on the bed, dead. A baby lay in a crib in the same room. Dr. Marten looked at the woman first, while a policeman told him the story.

The family who lived here consisted of the father and

mother, two older children, and the baby. That morning the father had left home for work at seven o'clock. Later, one of the older children noticed a faint odor of gas. Going into his mother's room he found her lying in bed. He shook her, but she would not move. He had run outside, leaving the door open and calling for help. A policeman had come, found an open gas jet in the room and turned it off. Then he had called for the medical examiner. The policeman told Dr. Marten that obviously the woman had been overcome by gas.

Marten looked at her and shook his head in doubt. There was none of the cherry red discoloration that often went with carbon monoxide.

Suddenly Dr. Marten thought of the child in the crib. He spun away from the woman's body and bent over the baby. It was still breathing, but with difficulty. "Get the oxygen!" he told the ambulance attendants who had come with him. "Quick!" He lifted the baby and ran with it into another room near an open window.

When he was sure the baby would live, Dr. Marten went back to examine the woman's body more closely. It seemed very strange that gas would kill a grown woman but not a baby in the same room. As he examined the woman, it seemed even stranger. There was no pink discoloration of the skin, but on the back of her neck there were eight small bruises. Dr. Marten put his hands on the woman's throat as if to choke her. His fingertips matched the bruises on the back of her neck.

"I want an autopsy," Marten said. "And a very careful one."

Science Catches the Criminal

The autopsy revealed just what he had expected. There was no carbon monoxide in the woman's blood or lungs. So she had already stopped breathing before gas entered the room. Also, the bruises went deep under her skin. And the hyoid bone was crushed. This is a small, horseshoe-shaped bone located just above the Adam's apple. When death is caused by choking or a fierce blow upon the throat, this bone is very likely to be broken.

Confronted with the evidence, the husband confessed. He'd had an argument with his wife and strangled her. Then he had put her body back on the bed, turned on the gas, and walked out, leaving his baby son in the crib beside his dead mother.

"If ever a man deserved to be hanged," Dr. Marten said later, "that one did." But if he himself had not noticed the color of the mother's body, if he had been a little slower to care for the baby, the baby would have died. It would have had carbon monoxide in its lungs. And if there had been no autopsy on the mother, the killer might well have gone free.

Some Light Poison

It was a few years after World War II that a young couple came to London's Scotland Yard carrying a pot of stew. They were, obviously, both angry and frightened, saying they wanted to report an attempted murder, a double murder, by poison.

It was an odd story, but the police listened respectfully.

They knew from experience that almost anything could be true.

The young man—not long out of the army—and his wife lived in a rented apartment on the second floor of a private home. The landlord was an old man who hated having anyone else in his house. Time after time he'd asked the young couple to leave. But since so many buildings had been destroyed during the war, housing was under the control of the government. The landlord then could not evict his tenants without reason.

For their part, the young couple did not think much of the landlord. He had eleven cats. The building not only smelled of cats, but some of them howled at night. Yet the couple stayed on simply because they could not find another place to live.

One day the wife came home from shopping to find the door to her upstairs apartment open. She went in, and there was the old landlord bending over a pot of stew she'd left cooking. "What are you doing in here?" she demanded.

He seemed excited. He stammered, "I—I smelled something burning. So I—I came up to look. You'd left this—this stew on the stove and—and it had boiled over."

That night when the couple had the stew for dinner, it tasted terrible. Even so, they ate a little of it. And both got sick.

Now they had brought the remains to Scotland Yard to be tested for poison.

The police were doubtful, but it was their job to check. The pot of stew was turned over to a chemist.

Science Catches the Criminal

At that time a thorough test for an unknown poison might take three weeks or even more. The chemist set to work, checking for one poison after another without success. At the same time he was haunted by a faint odor that came from the stew. He should, he thought, know what it was. And if he knew the poison he was looking for, then the tests would be easy. But days passed, and he kept working.

One night the chemist was awakened by his wife. Both she and the baby had colds; she wanted him to get up and give the baby a dose of medicine called cascara. The chemist got out of bed, stumbled into the bathroom, opened the cascara bottle, and suddenly shouted, "That's it!"

To his startled wife, the chemist explained: the pot of stew he had been studying for days smelled of cascara! The next day tests proved him right. And faced with this evidence, the landlord confessed. He had not wanted to harm the young couple; but he had wanted them to think they were being poisoned so they would leave his house. He had poured a whole bottle of cascara into their stew. Eaten, it would not have killed the young couple, but it would have made them sick.

A few years later the same chemist who had unraveled the Mystery of the Poisoned Stew was faced with an even odder situation. An old lady toddled into Scotland Yard carrying a cup of tea. Her husband, she said, had tried to poison her.

How did she know? Well, that morning her husband had gotten up early, made the tea, and brought her a cup while she was still in bed. In forty years of married life this was the first time he had done such a thing. So he must be trying to poison her.

This time the chemist found a quicker solution. He put the tea on the floor and the office cat drank it, without harm. Shaking her head, the old lady went home, happy but still puzzled.

9

THE LINDBERGH
KIDNAPPING

The World's Most Famous Baby

At about ten o'clock on the night of March 1, 1932, Mrs. Charles Lindbergh entered the room where her baby son was supposed to be sleeping. The baby's crib was empty. The window beyond the crib was partially open, a cold wind blowing in. On the nearby radiator lay a sealed envelope.

So began what newspapers referred to as "the world's most horrifying crime." Before the case was solved (there are still mysterious elements about it), it would involve some of the most brilliant scientific detection in the history of crime. Unfortunately, it would also include some of the very worst.

Back in the spring of 1927 Charles Lindbergh, a tall, rather shy young man, had flown an airplane called *The Spirit of St. Louis* across the Atlantic, alone. Today planes drone across the ocean like automobiles along a highway,

144

but in that spring of 1927 Charles Lindbergh was the first man ever to fly nonstop from New York to Paris.

Overnight Lindbergh became an international hero. When he married Anne Morrow, daughter of the American ambassador to Mexico, it was international news. When their first child was born and named Charles Augustus Lindbergh, Jr., his picture appeared in the newspapers of five continents, "The world's most famous baby."

This was the baby, twenty months old, who was stolen from his crib on the cold night of March 1, 1932.

The Lindberghs had chosen their home because of its privacy. It was on a winding dirt road, about three miles from the town of Hopewell, New Jersey, and the Hopewell police were the first to arrive. State troopers followed soon after. In the soft clay beneath the window of the baby's second-floor room they found marks where a ladder had been placed. Seventy feet away they found a crude, home-made ladder with one rung broken. It seemed obvious that ladder had been used to reach the baby's window; probably the one rung had broken when the kidnapper came down, carrying the extra weight of the child.

In their excitement dozens of policemen handled the ladder. Several times they made sure it fitted into the marks beneath the window—and in doing so they effectively rubbed out any fingerprints the kidnapper might have left.

Inside the house, Colonel Lindbergh had been much more careful. He did not even touch the envelope laying on the radiator until a fingerprint expert had arrived. But the envelope held no prints. Carefully then it was slit open and the note taken out. It read:

Science Catches the Criminal

Dear Sir

Have 50000$ ready 25000$ in 20$ bills 15000$ in 10$ bills and 10000$ in 5$ billsAfter 2-4 days we will inform you were to deliver the mony We warn you for making anyding public or for notify the police The child is in gut care

Indication for all letters are singnature and three holes

It was a curious signature and one Colonel Lindbergh would never forget. There were two interlocked circles, both outlined in blue. Inside the elipse where the circles overlapped there was a solid red oval. Three square holes had been punched in the paper, one in each part of the design.

But there were no fingerprints anywhere on the note.

If Colonel Lindbergh had opened the ransom note when he first found the baby missing, he might have heeded its warning not to call the police. Now it was too late. Not only had the police arrived, but newspapers all over the country were setting up enormous headlines for their morning editions.

Lindbergh Baby Kidnapped

Long before daylight reporters were crowding the Lindbergh estate. And when the newspapers appeared, what followed was enough, one reporter wrote, to make one ashamed of the human race. Literally by the thousands people headed for the Lindbergh home. They came not to help

146

—there was no help they could give—but to stand and stare and gossip. They blocked the road with their cars, and got stuck in the ditches. The police could not handle the crowds. Peddlers began to sell hotdogs and cold drinks, turning the whole thing into a kind of gruesome circus.

For Colonel and Mrs. Lindbergh the one thing that mattered was the safe return of their baby. Since his historic flight to Paris, Lindbergh had made a great deal of money. Besides, Mrs. Lindbergh's father was one of the richest men in the country. The $50,000 could be raised without problems.

But how could they contact the kidnappers? Or how could the kidnappers contact them when the roads were jammed for miles around and the police had set up an entire telephone substation in the Lindbergh garage?

Through the newspapers Colonel Lindbergh announced that he was willing to pay the ransom. But one day followed another and there was no word from the kidnappers. There were letters and calls from persons who claimed to be the kidnappers; they would return the child once they had been given the money. None of these, however, carried the curious signature of the original ransom note or offered any proof that the writers actually had the child.

This was the situation when on March 5, Dr. John Francis Condon, who had never met or even seen Colonel Lindbergh, decided to write a letter.

Dr. Condon was a seventy-two-year-old retired schoolteacher. He lived in the Bronx, one of the boroughs of New York City, and for a number of years he had written

letters to the Bronx *Home News* on a variety of subjects.
Now, on the night of March 5, he wrote to the paper:

> I offer all I can scrape together so a loving mother
> may again have her child and Colonel Lindbergh may
> know that the American people are grateful for the
> honor bestowed upon them by his pluck and daring.
>   Let the kidnappers know that no testimony of mine,
> or information coming from me, will be used against
> them. I offer $1,000.00 which I have saved from my
> salary (all my life savings), in addition to the sug-
> gested $50,000. I am ready at my own expense to go
> anywhere, also to give the kidnappers the extra money
> and never utter their names to anyone . . .

The Bronx *Home News* was a small paper. Practically
no one outside the Bronx ever saw it. The chance that anyone connected with the kidnapping would see Dr. Condon's
letter was very slim indeed.

The letter appeared on March 8. On March 9 Dr. Condon had several lectures to make and it was almost 10:00
P.M. when he came home. His wife had put the day's mail
on the mantel in the dining room. One of the letters was
addressed to:

Mr Doctor John F. Condon
2974 Decatur Avenue
New York

Dr. Condon cut open the envelope and as he read, his hands
began to shake.

148

The Lindbergh Kidnapping

Dear Sir: If you are willing to act as go-between in Lindbergh case pleace follow stricly instruction. Handel incloced letter *personaly* to Mr Lindbergh . . . As soon we found out the Press or Police is notifyed everything are cansell and it will be a further delay.

Affter you get the mony from Mr Lindbergh put these 3 words in the *New York American*

MONY IS REDY

Affter notise we will give you further instruction . . . Be at home every night between 6-12 . . .

The long envelope addressed to Dr. Condon also held a small envelope. On it was written, "Dear Sir: Please handel incloced letter to Colonal Lindbergh . . ."

His knees still shaking, Dr. Condon went to the telephone and called the Lindbergh home. He talked first with one policeman, then another. At last he got Lindbergh himself on the phone and read the letter, explaining there was another letter, addressed to Lindbergh, which he had not read.

"Open it and read it," Lindbergh told him.

Dr. Condon tore open the envelope. The note inside said, "Dear Sir: Mr. Condon may act as go-between . . . Affter we have the mony in hand we will tell you where to find your boy . . ."

There had been other letters from unknown persons demanding ransom. In all probability this was just another phony. Wearily Lindbergh asked, "Is that all?"

"Well," Dr. Condon said, "there's an odd looking picture . . . one circle cutting through another. And some holes in the paper."

Lindbergh's voice was suddenly excited. "Where are you? I'll come right away."

"No," Dr. Condon said. "You have enough to do. I'll come where you are."

Condon did not drive, and a friend took him to the Lindbergh home. It was long after midnight when they arrived, but the Lindberghs were waiting for them. Together they studied the note, and made plans. The one thing of importance was to get the baby back safely. To do this, they must act secretly: if the newspapers learned that Dr. Condon was acting for Lindbergh, then reporters would follow him in such numbers they would frighten off the kidnappers. So Condon needed some name that would be recognized by the kidnappers but not by the public.

"If you take my initials, J. F. C.," the old man told Lindbergh, "and pronounce them in a hurry, you have Jafsie."

And so the ad that appeared in the *New York American* read:

MONEY IS READY. JAFSIE

That night at a little after seven the phone in Dr. Condon's home rang. When he answered a man's voice, deep, with a heavy German accent said, "Is this Dr. John F. Condon?"

"Yes."

"Did you get my letter with the signature, the circles and holes?" The word *signature* was pronounced *singnature*.

"Yes."

150

The Lindbergh Kidnapping

Speaking with a German accent the man told Condon he must stay at home every night between six and twelve. He would get more instructions. He must follow these exactly or the whole thing would be off.

At this point Dr. Condon heard another voice. He heard it clearly, speaking it Italian, a language the doctor understood. It said, *"Sta zitto!"* meaning, "Shut up!"

Again there was a pause. The first voice said to Condon, "We will get in touch with you again." The phone went dead.

The very next night Condon received a special delivery letter. Signed with the rings and holes, it directed the old man to go immediately to an abandoned frankfurter stand on Jerome Avenue and to look under a large rock he would find there.

Dr. Condon didn't yet have the money; the ransom note had stated that it must be paid in certain denominations and Lindbergh was still getting it together. But Condon was glad of a chance to make personal contact with the kidnappers.

Again his friend drove him. He found the rock and under it a note that instructed him to walk across the street and follow an iron fence to 233rd Street.

Condon did, alone now. When he reached 233rd Street he found there was a park on one side, a cemetery on the other behind the fence. There were no houses in sight and distant street lights gave only a pale glimmer.

The old man waited. He was about to give up when, suddenly, someone spoke to him from inside the fence. "Did you get it, the money?"

"No. I can't bring the money until I know the baby is safe."

From inside the fence came a noise that might have been a footstep, or a dead limb falling from a tree. Instantly the man opposite Condon leaped, caught the top of the fence, and swung himself over. He jumped to the sidewalk, raced across the street and into the park. Condon ran heavily after him. Suddenly they were face to face in the darkness. "You sent the cops!" the man said.

"No. The cemetery may have guards, but I didn't send anyone."

The man made no attempt to hide his face and though it was dark in the park, Condon could see that he had deep-set eyes, a long, narrow chin. "You should have brought the money," he said after a moment.

Condon repeated that he could not bring the money until he knew the baby was safe. The kidnapper shook his head. He assured Condon the baby was safe, but it could not be returned without the ransom. There were others in the gang. They would kill him if he tried to return the child without getting the money. However, he would send a token to prove they had the baby. He would send the pajamas the child had been wearing when stolen.

On this point the kidnapper kept his word. The pajamas were mailed to Condon's house. After them came other letters and calls. The kidnappers would not give up the child before they got the money. But in exchange for the money they would give Dr. Condon a note telling exactly where to find the baby.

Lindbergh accepted these terms because he had no

152

choice. On the night of April 2 Dr. Condon met once more with the kidnapper. Condon handed over the money and the kidnapper gave him a note. It said the child would be found on board a small boat between Horseneck Beach and Gay Head near Elizabeth Island.

For two days Lindbergh searched for his child, using planes and boats. There was no sign of the baby. Dr. Condon put new ads in the papers begging the kidnappers to get in touch with him. There was no answer. A month passed, five weeks, six weeks, and no word.

The Most Horrifying Crime

It was purely by accident that a man named William Allen on May 12 discovered the body of a child in some woods about five miles from the Lindbergh estate. The body had been buried in a shallow grave, but now spring rains had washed away most of dirt. Although the body was largely decayed, there was no doubt of the identity. The child's face, that had been pressed into the earth, was still recognizable. An autopsy gave the official cause of death: "The child died of a fractured skull caused by external violence."

Exactly how the skull had been fractured, it was impossible to say, but the blow had been violent. Possibly the kidnapper had struck the child while it was still in its crib, making sure it did not cry out when moved. Or the baby may have been dropped when the rung of the ladder broke. But one thing was certain: the baby had died at the time of the kidnapping or very soon thereafter. Probably the kidnapper had carried the corpse of the child directly from the Lindbergh house to the place where it was buried.

While there was still a chance the baby might be recovered safely, the police had restrained their search. Now there was no need for restraint. But what did they have to work with?

There was the homemade ladder on which more than 125 fingerprints had been found. But these were all of police and reporters.

There were the handwritten ransom notes.

There was the fact that Dr. Condon had met face to face with the kidnapper and might be able to identify him, even though the meetings had been in the dark.

Also, the serial numbers of all the ransom money had been listed. Some of these bills were of an old-fashioned type, slightly larger than new bills and easy to identify. However, a great many bills of this type were still in circulation.

It was the money and old-fashioned police work that located the kidnapper. But it was the ladder and an almost incredible piece of scientific detection that did the most to convict him.

After the body was found months passed with no real progress by the police. Banks all over the country had been alerted to be on the lookout for the ransom money, and gradually bills began to turn up. Now and then a bank could trace the money to the depositor; but always this was a store, or someone who had received the money in change and could easily prove that he or she had nothing to do with the kidnapping.

Most of the identified bills were in the New York area. And slowly it became evident that more were being spent in the Bronx than in any other part of the city.

Police reasoned that the kidnappers must certainly have used an automobile. So every filling station in the New York area was given a list of the ransom bills and told to be on the lookout.

In September of 1934, approximately two-and-a-half years after the baby had been kidnapped and killed, a dark blue Dodge sedan stopped for gas at a filling station on the corner of Lexington Avenue and 127th Street in New York. The driver was a lean, athletic-looking man who spoke with a German accent. He paid for his gas with an old-fashioned ten dollar bill.

"You don't see many of these any more," the filling station operator said.

"Ya," the driver said. "I have only a few left."

He took his change and drove off. But as he did the filling station operator remembered the police request to be on the lookout for such bills. So he took out a pencil and wrote the license number of the Dodge sedan on the back of the bill.

A police check showed that this bill was part of the ransom money. Another check showed that the license plate was registered in the name of Bruno Richard Hauptmann, 1279 East 222nd Street, The Bronx.

When arrested, Hauptmann had several of the ransom

bills in his pocket. Buried under the floor of his garage police found another $13,760 of the money.

Even so, Hauptmann swore that he'd had nothing to do with the kidnapping. His story was that back in 1932 he'd been in business with man named Isidor Fisch. Like Hauptmann, Fisch was German-born. His health was poor and he'd told Hauptmann that he wanted to go back to Germany for a visit. Before leaving he gave Hauptmann a large cardboard box to keep for him. Fisch had died while in Germany and the box had stayed in Hauptmann's closet for months, forgotten. But the roof leaked and the box got wet. When Hauptmann went to move it, the box fell apart and he saw the money. Since Fisch was dead, Hauptmann said, he'd just decided to keep the money.

Hauptmann stuck to his story and nothing could shake it. Dr. Condon was sure that Hauptmann was the man he'd met, but Hauptmann merely shook his head. Mistaken identities were quite common.

There were handwriting experts who would testify that all fourteen of the ransom notes had been written by Hauptmann. But there were also experts who would testify they had not been written by him. The police knew from experience that it was almost impossible to prove anything by handwriting.

From the first most police had felt certain that one man could not have done the kidnapping alone. They believed it was the work of a gang. But try as they would, they could find no evidence that Richard Hauptmann had ever been connected with any gang.

Hauptmann's lawyer sincerely believed his client was

innocent. He felt sure that when the case came to trial he would be acquitted.

The Xylotomist

There was, however, one bit of evidence that even Hauptmann himself did not know about. It had been acquired by some of the most brilliant and painstaking scientific work in the history of crime.

When the story of the Lindbergh kidnapping first broke in the newspapers, a man named Arthur Koehler was working for the government Forest Service at a laboratory in Madison, Wisconsin. Koehler was a xylotomist, a scientist who studied the growth patterns and cellular structure of various kinds of wood. When he first read of the kidnapping and the homemade ladder which had been used, Koehler wrote to Colonel Lindbergh. If he could study the ladder, Koehler said, he might be of help in tracing it.

Hundreds, probably thousands, of other persons also wrote to the Lindberghs at this time. The letters were opened by police or servants, put aside and forgotten.

In February of 1933, almost a year after the kidnapping, the New Jersey police asked the Forest Service for help. The Forest Service immediately sent for their top expert, Arthur Koehler.

Koehler did not look like a detective. He was of average height, a little plump, his eyes a bit squinted. Now for four days he looked at the ladder, studying it piece by piece, inch by inch.

Science Catches the Criminal

The ladder had been made in three separate sections that could be fitted together to increase the length. Koehler saw these were made of four different kinds of wood: second growth southern pine, Douglas fir, Ponderosa pine, and a few pieces of birch.

To study it more closely, Koehler took the ladder apart, numbering each piece. In one of the pieces—to Koehler it was #16—he found four nail holes. They had been made by old-fashioned square nails. These had not been driven straight into the wood, but at slightly differing angles. And there was no rust around the holes.

"Wherever this piece of wood was used before," Koehler told the police, "it was inside a shelter of some kind. It's never been exposed to rain. If we could find the piece of wood it was nailed to, with square nail holes matching the angles of these, we'd know it exactly. There's not one chance in a million there could be another four square holes, matching these angles exactly."

But how to find that piece of wood?

Koehler began to study the ladder not inch by inch, but by tiny fractions of inches, under a microscope. Each one of the pine rungs had been smoothed down with a plane. To Koehler, peering through his microscope, the marks of the plane were as unique as fingerprints. They had been made with a hand plane using a dull blade.

Unless the blade had been much used or sharpened in the meanwhile, Koehler would be able to identify it. But like the nail holes, this information was of no use in tracing the ladder to its source.

The ladder rails were of southern pine. Studying them

158

under the microscope, Koehler found a series of tiny grooves. These ran through the tops of microscopic waves made by the planing mill where the lumber was originally dressed. These waves were exactly eighty-six hundredths of an inch apart. The grooves meant that one of the knives at this mill had some nick or irregularity in it, a flaw so small it could not be seen except under a magnifying glass. Also, Koehler could tell there had been six knives in the cutting head of the planer. The space between the waves told him the plank had been fed through the mill at a rate of 230 feet-per-minute.

Now to find that mill.

Southern pine grows chiefly in the Atlantic coastal states. But there were 1,600 planing mills in that area that used this type of lumber.

Koehler wrote to every one of them asking for basic information about the size of lumber they processed, the type of cutting head, the speed of the pulleys. From their answers he eliminated all but twenty-five. These he asked to send him samples of wood.

From the M.G. & J.J. Dorn Company in South Carolina Koehler got a sample that matched the ladder rail in every way except one: the spacing of the grooves on one side was wrong. Koehler hurried to the mill to talk with its officials. Why yes, one of them told him, there had been a time, starting back in September, 1929, when they had used a pulley that wasn't standard. No one remembered just how long they had used it, but it had been replaced after a year or so.

The old pulley was still around. The mill officials were

159

willing to help. And when the old pulley was put on, the lumber passing through the cutter head matched that of the kidnap ladder in every particular.

So now Koehler knew the mill from which the lumber had come. But where had it gone from here?

Koehler knew there would be microscopic changes almost day by day in the marks made by the mill's cutter head. So he would be able to identify the exact shipment of lumber, if he could find it.

He started with the mill's shipping records. There had been carload after carload to lumberyards all over the East. Koehler decided to concentrate on those in the New York area. One of these was in the Bronx and Koehler went there. The manager shook his head. They had bought one carload from the Dorn Company, he said. But it was all sold and they had no records of who had bought it.

The New Jersey police had assigned a detective to work with Koehler. Together they went to one lumberyard after another. Sometimes there was lumber from the Dorn Mill on hand; sometimes all the lumber was gone, but records showed who had bought at least part of it. Koehler and his detective went to work. In one place the lumber had been used to build a doghouse; in another it was part of a garage; in another an attic. By now the look of the wood he sought was engraved in Koehler's mind. He needed only a quick glance through a pocket magnifying glass to know. None of it was what he wanted.

The search kept on. In one place the lumber had all been sold, but as Koehler was leaving the manager remembered they had used part of it themselves. It did not match the image in Koehler's mind. Even so, it gave him an idea.

He went back to the lumberyard in the Bronx that had received a shipment from the Dorn Company but sold it all. Was it possible, Koehler asked, they might have used a little bit of it themselves?

The manager called in his assistant and suddenly one of them remembered. They had used part of this lumber to build some bins. Minutes later Arthur Koehler knew that this part of his hunt had come to an end. Part of the lumber in the kidnap ladder had come from this particular yard. It had come from a shipment received on December 1, 1931, just three months before the kidnapping.

But there the trail ended. The lumber had been sold for cash, piece by piece, and so there was no record of who had bought it. No one in the lumberyard could remember a single sale of this particular lumber.

(Later it would be learned that Hauptmann had worked in this lumberyard at the time the Dorn Company shipment had arrived. But at this time no one assigned to the Lindbergh case had ever even heard of Bruno Richard Hauptmann.)

Koehler did not give up. He started now to trace another bit of lumber from the ladder. Before he got far, the filling station operator had jotted down Hauptmann's license number on the back of the ransom bill and he was arrested.

So the case came to court with Hauptmann and his lawyers feeling certain he would be acquitted. They had the story of Isidor Fisch to explain the kidnap money. They could claim that Dr. Condon, an old man, might easily be mistaken about a person he had seen only twice, both times in the dark. They had experts to swear Hauptmann had not written the ransom notes. And Hauptmann's wife testified that he had been with her the night of the kidnapping.

Then the prosecution called Arthur Koehler to the witness stand.

Koehler explained how he had traced the ladder rails to a lumberyard in the Bronx—the same lumberyard where it was now known Hauptmann had worked. But this was not all. Koehler told how he and a police detective had searched Hauptmann's home after his arrest. In the garage they found a number of carpentry tools. One of these was the blade of a hand plane, dull and unused for a long time.

Koehler now brought out some greatly enlarged photographs of microscopic studies. With these he showed that it was this very same blade that had been used to plane the rungs of the ladder. The ladder had been made with Hauptmann's tools.

Still Koehler was not through. He showed the rung of the ladder that had four holes made by square nails. He told how, in searching Hauptmann's home, he and the detective had gone into the attic. There they found where a piece of the rough flooring had been sawed off. The sawdust was still on the attic floor. Under the microscope Koehler was able to tell that the ladder rung and the sawed board were part of the same bit of timber.

And still he was not through. This part of his evidence was so technical that some of the jurors might doubt it. There was still more. In Hauptmann's attic Koehler and the detective found a board with four holes made by old-fashioned square nails. Koehler placed the ladder rung over the attic board. He took four square nails and put them in the holes. They fitted perfectly, the angle of every one absolutely the same.

The kidnap ladder had not only been made with at least one of Hauptmann's tools, part of the ladder had come from his attic.

The jury handed down a verdict of guilty.

After it was all over Hauptmann's lawyer sputtered in anger, "We'd have won an acquittal—if it hadn't been for that guy Koehler. A xylotomist! The word isn't even in most dictionaries!"

There were many people, including many police, who believed that Richard Hauptmann could not have staged the kidnapping alone. Who was it Dr. Condon had heard over the phone speaking Italian?

No one ever learned. On the night of April 3, 1936, Bruno Richard Hauptmann went to the electric chair. He still maintained that he was innocent.

10

CRIME AND SCIENCE

Today and Tomorrow

Today a chemist searching for an unknown poison would face an even more difficult problem than the Scotland Yard expert with the poisoned stew. Within the past few years pharmaceutical houses have developed literally thousands of new drugs, many of them poisons. It might well take a year or more to make the tests necessary for all of them. If these tests had to be made on the body of a murder victim, it would be impossible. Forensic scientists say there simply is not enough tissue in the human body for all the tests.

On the other hand, if there is reason to suspect a particular poison, then—in most cases but not all—the test is relatively simple. And the scientist is rarely faced with total mystery when he and the police work together. It is this combination of forensic scientist and police detective that often runs down the criminal. Take the case of Dr. Carl Coppolino.

Coppolino was a medical doctor, a specialist in anesthesiology. But he had retired while still young because, he said, of a heart attack. After that he lived on the income of his wife Carmela, also a doctor, and on a very handsome disability income from insurance. He and his wife moved to Sarasota, Florida. And there one day in 1965 Carmela died, suddenly.

Coppolino said his wife's death was due to a heart attack. The local doctor, who knew Coppolino was a doctor and something of a specialist in heart problems, took his word for it and signed the death certificate. Carmela's body was sent back to New Jersey, her former home, for burial. And almost immediately Dr. Carl Coppolino married again, a wealthy young widow.

This might have been the end of the matter, had it not been for another widow. This one was neither as young nor as rich as the second Mrs. Coppolino. Her name was Marge Farber and she went to the Sarasota police with a strange story.

Mrs. Farber and her husband, Colonel Farber, had once been neighbors of the Coppolinos in New Jersey. Mrs. Farber and Carl Coppolino began a love affair. Carl became jealous of the colonel and, Marge Farber said, murdered him. She knew because she watched the whole thing. Coppolino gave her husband an injection of some drug that was supposed to kill him. When it did not act fast enough, Coppolino took a bed pillow and smothered the now unconscious colonel.

As to the death of Carmela Coppolino, Marge Farber knew nothing—except that Carmela had never had heart trouble.

The police began a quiet investigation that lasted for

165

months. Then Dr. Carl Coppolino was indicted for murder in both New Jersey and in Florida.

The New Jersey trial was held first, and Coppolino was found not guilty. His attorney convinced the jury that Marge Farber, jealous because her lover had married a younger woman after Carmela's death, had lied about the whole affair.

Now came the Florida trial, but most persons believed it would be a waste of time. If Coppolino had been acquitted for the murder of Colonel Farber, despite an eyewitness, how could he be convicted of killing his wife when there was no witness and no knowledge, so far as anyone knew, of how she actually died? But the Florida trial showed what could be done when police and scientists worked together.

The police quickly learned that when Carl and Carmela moved to Florida, Carmela had failed her Florida medical examination. She could no longer practice and this put an end to her income. The police also learned that the insurance companies paying Carl $22,000 a year were beginning to believe his heart trouble was faked. Carl also knew this, and that his income might stop. He needed money. It was at this time he met the rich young widow who made it plain she would be willing to marry him, if he were not already married to Carmela. Carl now took out an extra $65,000 insurance on Carmela's life.

After Carmela's death Carl had told neighbors that an autopsy had proved she died of a heart attack. The police learned there had never been an autopsy—because Carl had refused to have one.

There was one other item. Shortly before Carmela's death, Carl acquired a supply of a drug called succinylcholine chloride. This was a drug with which Coppolino was well acquainted, having frequently used it in his work as an anesthetist. Used in this way, it paralyzed muscles during an operation and kept them from trembling. But a large dose would also paralyze the muscles of the lungs, bringing death.

There was another peculiar and interesting thing about this drug. Injected into the human body it quickly broke down into its component parts. In doing this the drug, as such, disappeared. Many doctors believed that this was a perfect murder weapon since no known test could discover it in the human body.

This was as far as the police could go. Now the work was up to the forensic scientists.

Carmela's body was dug up and sent to the laboratory of Dr. Milton Helpern, the New York City Medical Examiner. Dr. Helpern himself did the autopsy, working day after day. At the Florida trial his testimony proved two points: one, Carmela had been in good health; she had not died of a heart attack. And second, she had been given an injection into her left buttock shortly before her death. Dr. Helpern had not only found the needle puncture, he had made incisions to show the exact depth. All this he had photographed with color slides that were shown to the shocked jury. What the injection was, Dr. Helpern did not try to say.

The prosecution now called Dr. Joseph Umberger. As the toxicologist in Dr. Helpern's office it had been his job to find and identify any poison in the body of Carmela Coppolino.

From Dr. Helpern's work, Umberger knew that Carmela had been given an injection of some kind just before her death. From the police work he knew this might be succinylcholine chloride. And from his own work he knew that no method had yet been devised to find this drug in the human body.

Dr. Umberger set out to devise such a method. He worked for six months with tissue from Carmela's brain, liver, kidneys, and other organs. If succinylcholine chloride broke down and no longer existed as a unit in the human body, then he must find the parts, or some part of the drug, and in such quantities that this could not have entered her body except by an injection of the poison.

Dr. Umberger described himself as an "old-fashioned" chemist. He worked with Bunsen burners and test tubes such as might have been found in nineteenth-century laboratories. But he also worked with the newest of instruments. By heating, Dr. Umberger changed some of the substances in Carmela's body from solid to gas. As a gas, this would burn. Using the spectograph—the same instrument that has been used in airplane accidents to discover the tiniest bit of explosive among the wreckage—Dr. Umberger found quantities of succinic acid, one of the components of succinylcholine chloride.

Coppolino's lawyer waved his hand and jeered. Minute quantities of succinic acid are present in every brain, he said.

Patiently Dr. Umberger explained. There are two types

of succinic acid. One the chemists refer to as "bound." By this they mean it is tied to the proteins and possibly other substances in human tissue. But there is another form of succinic acid, "unbound." Dr. Umberger referred to it as "store bought." This was the type he had found, and this could not have reached Carmela's brain except by poison.

For two and a half days Dr. Umberger sat on the witness stand. Most of this time Coppolino's lawyer badgered and shouted at him. But Umberger was not to be shaken. He was a scientist. He knew exactly what he had done and what he had found. His testimony convinced the jury.

Carl Coppolino was sent to prison for life.

Tomorrow?

The principles of the spectograph Dr. Umberger used to find succinic acid in Carmela Coppolino's body have been known for a half century or more. Modern techniques have made the device even more sensitive. In the war on crime, science is constantly contributing new weapons.

Police departments as well as industry are making increased use of computers. As sound spectrograms become more accurate and simplified, a national computerized file of voice prints may join such a file of fingerprints. If it becomes possible to identify a person as accurately by his blood as by his fingerprints—as now seems possible—there may be a computerized blood file. Then any police station in the country could, within minutes, absolutely identify any wanted individual whose blood, voice, or fingerprints was on record.

Police are already considering combining the computer with the TV camera to identify stolen automobiles. A television camera set up alongside a highway might photograph the license plates of passing cars. This information might be fed automatically into a computer, identifying within moments any plate that had been reported stolen.

Cameras in satellites circling the earth have already been able to locate hidden fields of poppies and other drug-producing plants.

Veteran police officers often say that "Identification is 90 per cent of the problem." If Dr. John Condon had been able to produce a recognizable likeness of Bruno Richard Hauptmann, it is very likely he would have been caught much sooner. Police artists have often tried to draw, from the description given by a witness, the picture of a criminal. Now there are several devices that make this much easier and more accurate than in the past. These go by such names as Mug-a-Minute, or Identi-Kit. Basically they make use of predrawn or photographed features. These can be flashed one at a time, or several together, upon a screen. The witness can select the hair, eyes, nose, and so on that most resemble the wanted man, then put them together. Sometimes this has produced a remarkable resemblance, and a quick arrest.

One of the most fantastic new devices is called Nuclear Activation Analysis, the product of cooperation between the Atomic Energy Commission and various industries. This works on the principle that every element, bombarded by atoms, gives off its own characteristic radiation. This is so sensitive that a teaspoon of arsenic can be identified in ten tank cars of water. A fragment of paint on a burglar's tool so small as to be invisible to the human eye can be matched precisely to the door or window from which it was broken—and this has been done in at least one case, sending the burglar to jail.

It is unlikely, of course, that scientific advances will ever put an end to crime. But it is certain that the scientists of the future will make the criminal's life ever more difficult.

INDEX

172

Index

174